The Nurse Practitioner:
Real-world Research in A&E

The Nurse Practitioner: Real-world Research in A&E

Brian Dolan

MSc (Oxon), MSc (Lond), BSc (Hons), RMN, RGN, CHSM
Nursing Research Fellow, King's A&E Primary Care Service,
London; Editor – *Emergency Nurse*

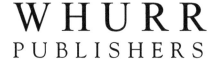

WHURR PUBLISHERS

© 2000 Whurr Publishers Ltd
First published 2000 by
Whurr Publishers Ltd
19b Compton Terrace
London N1 2UN England, and 325 Chestnut Street, Philadelphia PA 19106, USA

Reprinted 2001

British Library Cataloguing in Publication Data
A catalogue record for this book is available from the British Library.

ISBN 1 86156 141 5

Printed in the UK by Athenæum Press Ltd, Gateshead, Tyne & Wear

Contents

Acknowledgements

I would like especially to thank the following people:

The Emergency Nurse Practitioners and staff at the pilot site, who were so generous with their time, energy and commitment to supporting this study. This book is dedicated to the excellence of their care.

Dr Hazel Hagger for her unflustered approach to supervision – it made for an enjoyable experience.

Dr Mike Walsh, Reader in Nursing at the University College of St Martin's for his generosity in sharing his experience of this specialized field of nursing.

Janet Marsden, Senior Lecturer, Manchester Metropolitan University, for helping to link my thinking between theory and practice.

Professor Jeremy Dale, Primary Care Unit, University of Warwick and Dr Edward Glucksman, A&E Consultant, King's College Hospital NHS Trust for all their ongoing support and encouragement over the years I have known them.

To Lynda and William for their love, support and ability to keep life in happy, healthy perspective.

Not least to South Thames NHS Executive, who generously funded this study through the provision of a South Thames Research Training Fellowship.

Brian Dolan

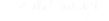

Preface

Nurse practitioners working in emergency care settings, such as accident and emergency departments and minor injury units, are perceived to offer equitable, accessible care that is patient centred. Studies that have compared them with other professionals, usually doctors, have found them to offer care that is safe, effective and efficient. What is less clear, however, is why nurse practitioners working in emergency care settings are so successful and popular with patients. The consultation process may offer some clues to answer this question.

This pilot study describes the methodological issues associated with researching nurse practitioner–patient consultations, and tests a range of research instruments designed to capture the process and content of these consultations and appraise patient satisfaction with them. After gaining informed consent, patients were asked to have their consultation with the nurse practitioner audiotaped. This was analysed using the Multi-dimensional Interaction Analysis research tool. Separate and different post-consultation questionnaires were completed by the patients and nurse practitioners in the study. An audit of the clinical content of the nurse practitioner records was also undertaken.

While, as this was a pilot study, no claims can be made about the data, it appears that the Multi-dimensional Interaction Analysis research tool and the patients' Medical Interview Satisfaction Scale are sufficiently robust for the main study. A semi-structured interview schedule may provide a richer source of data than the post-consultation questionnaire administered to nurse practitioners in the study. The audit of the clinical content of the nurse practitioner records also appears to be reliable and valid, but it does not fully reflect the amount of health education and advice given to patients by the nurse practitioners, suggesting that case note audits are an inadequate indicator of quality care. These methodological issues will be addressed before undertaking the larger doctoral study.

Chapter 1
Introduction

Nursing is simply a practice, but its practice is far from simple. While the conception of nursing lies in its Latin origins (*nutrire* meaning to nourish), it is also perceived as something that anyone can do. It is even somewhat pejoratively viewed as 'women's work' (Dolan 1993). Yet nursing is a complex, intellectually demanding, physically challenging role; one which is so subtle in its application that we sometimes only recognize how good it can be if we see or are subjected to poor quality care.

For nurses who work in emergency care settings, the subtlety of nursing practice can be masked by the array of biomedical high technology that is found there. The care, comfort and education services provided by a skilled nurse are more subtle and abstract to the patient than is a well-performed technological procedure (albeit often more valued than the latter), yet much of everyday experience in nursing is overlooked and taken for granted because it is skilful coping in the midst of an ongoing situation.

In its perceived simplicity, nursing is thus rendered invisible. Even such highly regarded feminist scholars as Ann Oakley noted this when she 'confessed' (her term) that during a '15 year career as a sociologist studying medical services', she had 'been particularly blind to the contribution made by nurses to health care' (Oakley 1984, p 24). It was some of this invisibility and its attendant consequences for the development of the nursing profession that was one of the driving forces behind this study.

The other driving force was an interest in a relatively new role in nursing, that of the emergency nurse practitioner (ENP). These are experienced clinical nurses who assess, investigate, diagnose, treat and discharge and/or refer patients without recourse to a medical practitioner. Their work has in many ways legitimized the surreptitious practice that had for years occurred in emergency care settings. For example, if a patient required an X-ray for an injured wrist, he or she was frequently sent for one by nurses despite the lack of an official sanction to do so. Sanction was often denied because of tribal feuds between health-care professionals that prevented the nurse from delivering high-quality care to the patient. Too often in health care, patients have been used as pawns in a game of professional chess in which giving ground has been seen as losing face instead of a means of improving care. The development of the ENP role in accident and emergency (A&E), and minor injury unit (MIU) settings, as well as elsewhere, has underlined the skills and expertise of nurses in delivering that care safely and effectively.

Since the beginning of the 1990s, the number of ENPs has grown considerably, yet, as will be seen in the selected literature review, studies of nurse practitioners have more often than not compared them with other professionals, usually junior doctors, rather than exploring what they do themselves. Metaphorically speaking, nurses and doctors are like apples and oranges – both are fruit, but there the similarities quickly come to an end. So it is with nurse practitioners and doctors – both are health-care professionals but with different cultures, emphases and backgrounds. As will be shown in the literature review, nurse practitioners are particularly successful in their role as they appear to offer a more equitable, accessible relationship, which is valued by patients. What has been sorely lacking in the literature, however, has been detailed studies seeking to understand why this is so.

While many of the studies that have looked at the ENP role have compared their ability with that of doctors to, for example, request and interpret X-rays (Meek et al 1995, Freij et al 1996) or administer medicines (Marshall et al 1997), and have in the process helped to establish their clinical safety and effectiveness, there are very few studies that have sought to answer the more difficult question 'Why are ENPs so popular with patients?'. Part of the secret of that popularity perhaps lies in that period 'behind the screens', to borrow Jocalyn Lawlor's (1991) evocative imagery, suggesting that when ENPs and patients are engaged in a consultation, the former are at their most successful and effective.

The consultation is, however, also the period in their practice when nurses are most invisible, and it is the combination of making the invisible visible and the fact that it is nurse practitioners who are delivering this care in emergency care settings that is the driving force behind this study.

During my early nursing career in mental health nursing, it was clear that the combination of mental health and general nursing skills could be most readily applied in an A&E department, where, amidst the high technology, human dramas in health care were being played out. At that time, however, nursing practice in A&E was relatively restricted, and patients could wait many hours to be seen by a medical practitioner before having relatively minor conditions such as a cut treated – ironically by a nurse, who knew what needed to be done anyway. It was, especially at that time, both an exciting and a demanding environment in which to practise the art and science of nursing.

Subsequently, for the first few months of my practice as a newly qualified general staff nurse, while absorbed in learning the craft of A&E nursing practice, the institutional restrictions imposed on nursing became obvious. Mental health nursing is to a greater extent imbued with a philosophy of 'the title of the person giving the care doesn't matter as much as being able to care for the person', highlighting within the situation in general nursing in A&E a waste of good resources and, more importantly, a cause of needless pain, suffering and delay for the patients.

Mental health nursing stresses the need to establish a rapport with patients and engage them in an interpersonal relationship. This can be extremely difficult with patients whose personalities are breaking or have broken down, as in the case of schizophrenia, or who are elated or deeply subdued, as in cases of mania and severe depression. Yet it was the development and use of these interpersonal skills that forged my interest in nurse–patient relationships. Personal observation and the literature made it apparent that nurses were seen as trustworthy by patients, who would reveal more of their condition to nurses than they would to doctors, doctors too often being seen as omnipotent and, rather unfairly, especially perhaps in mental health, somewhat patrician and distant.

Yet while doctors were given the credit for curing patients, nurses were given the boxes of chocolates for caring for them, and although this paints a rather arbitrary line between the two health-care professions that in practice rarely exists, it nonetheless graphically illustrates the fact that patients would publicly laud the doctors' skills, but privately value the nurses' ability to care for them and care about them as people when they were at their most frightened and vulnerable.

To use a clinical example, it was not the skilful insertion of an intravenous line by the doctor that mattered to the patient, but the nurse's ability to judge when the patient needed a hand held in comfort that determined quality care. Yet, once the screens around the bed or hospital trolley were pulled back, I frequently heard the patient say to relatives, 'They [the doctors] were very good, the injection (sic) didn't hurt much at all.' Nursing once more became invisible.

If nursing can be seen as a form of social justice in which those who are frightened, distressed and in pain can be given comfort, relief and succour, it is incumbent on researchers to try to explore not just what nurses do, but what nursing is. And if the nurse–patient consultation is at the heart of nursing, this is where it is best explored. In essence, this study is centred on the privatized and professional everyday working lives of a group of nurses, hence being about the things that are not usually considered worthy of investigation in nursing because they are so taken for granted. While the purpose of the pilot study that will be described in this book is metaphorically to test the road-worthiness of the research instruments, if the main study that follows is successful, it is to be hoped it will open up an under-explored dimension of nursing practice – a practice that remains far from simple.

Chapter 2
Literature review

Interest in the ENP concept has stimulated fertile debate in the field of health care in recent years, particularly in A&E and MIU settings. The ENP's role provides a relatively new minor injury and illness service complementary to that currently provided by medical staff. Clinical decisions made by ENPs, when comparing them with those made by medical practitioners, are shown to be safe and effective (Tye 1997). Patient satisfaction with ENP services is shown to be high, and patients also appreciate the more relaxed and equal style of consultation offered by nurse practitioners (Johnson 1993, Cooper & Robb 1996, Reveley 1998). However, beyond Stilwell et al's work (1987), which was set in a primary care setting, there is a gap in the UK literature in relation to the consultation behaviour of nurse practitioners. Research examining the consultation process between nurse practitioners and patients in emergency care settings is also particularly sparse.

This review of the literature will seek critically to analyse and evaluate selected published papers related to nurse practitioners working in emergency care settings. It will review the history of the nurse practitioner movement, consider papers that have examined the role development and clinical activities of ENPs, and examine the research available relating to consultations between doctors and patients, and nurses and patients. Based on this review, a range of questions relating to the process and content of consultations between nurse practitioners and patients in emergency care settings will be identified. In subsequent chapters, both the methodological theory and its practical application in the pilot study of the research relating to addressing these questions will be examined.

In undertaking this selected literature review, the following databases were utilized: the Royal College of Nursing (RCN) *Bibliography*, Medline (the *International Nursing Index* and *Index Medicus*), King's College London's *Libertas*, and the *Cumulative Index of Nursing and Allied Health Literature* (CINAHL). The following terms were entered into each database: 'nurse practitioner', 'emergency nurse', 'emergency nurse practitioner', 'emergency care', 'minor injuries', 'consultations', 'doctor–patient consultations' and 'nurse–patient consultations'. The literature reviewed stems predominantly from the UK, but there is much literature available from the USA. Much of the literature assessed relates to papers published in the 1980s or 90s; however, where appropriate, a number of seminal papers from the 1960s and 70s have been included.

Aims of the literature review

The aims of this literature review are:

- to outline the history of the nurse practitioner movement;
- to define the role of the ENP;
- to consider the clinical activities of ENPs;
- to examine studies looking at consultation processes between nurses and patients, and doctors and patients;
- to identify gaps in the literature and formulate questions that could be addressed by empirical investigation.

Historical development

The nurse practitioner movement (as it has become known) was founded in 1965 at the University of Colorado in Denver (Dunn 1997) by a nurse Loretta Ford and doctor John Silver, in an attempt to ease the critical shortage of primary care physicians in the mid-western area of the USA. The shortage arose partly as a result of the Vietnam War, but more specifically because doctors did not wish to work in relatively less affluent communities, which afforded them less income. The inception of the nurse practitioner role occurred in response to an increased awareness of inequalities in health care, partly, but not exclusively, brought about as a consequence of the shortage of doctors. The role was initiated via a feasibility project, the purpose of which was to determine whether nurses could provide better and more widely available health care for children (Mauksch 1987).

The ENP emerged in the mid-1970s in the USA in response to the increased use of American Emergency Rooms (ERs), which resulted from the increased specialization of physicians, the lower number of general medical practitioners, the inaccessibility of medical care, especially at nights and weekends, and the mobile nature of the American population (Geolet 1975, Hayden et al 1982). The clinical management of some patients with minor injuries by a nurse practitioner in the A&E department at Oldchurch Hospital, Romford, first attracted attention of the British nursing press in 1988 (Head 1988), and an in-house study of this scheme was published in 1989 (Morris et al 1989).

Read and George (1994), however, note that for a long period prior to this, nurses in MIUs, particularly in community hospitals and general practitioner (GP) hospitals, had in essence functioned as nurse practitioners, using their clinical judgement about whether to call in a doctor, send a patient to a major A&E department, something that Dale and Dolan (1996) found to be a relatively rare event, or treat a patient within agreed guidelines without a medical opinion being obtained.

In more recent years, a growing number of British hospital A&E departments have been employing ENPs, usually sisters/charge nurses with a number of years of experience in clinical practice. Unlike the situation in the USA, however, where all ENPs must undertake a Master's degree to be allowed to practise (Cole et al 1998), UK-trained ENPs may have undertaken anything from a 1-week course to a full 3-year honours BSc degree. Walsh (1997) believes that, in view of the high levels of responsibility carried by the nurse practitioners, anything less than the 2-year RCN Nurse Practitioner diploma seems inadequate unless the nurse is working in a very restricted field. Part of the problem with the nurse practitioner role is its definition, and this will be examined in the next section.

Defining the ENP role

Problems of definition abound, and the title 'nurse practitioner is much abused and is little understood by the service, and more importantly, by patients' (Casey 1996). Dale et al (1996) found that the 'term nurse practitioner was being used to describe a wide range of nursing roles'. They argued that the use of interchangeable terms and concepts is likely to lead to confusion during the commissioning of services, and called for a clearer understanding of terminology to enable clarity of understanding when service developments, such as the nurse practitioner role, are being negotiated between health service purchasers and providers.

The RCN A&E Nursing Association (Royal College of Nursing 1992) defines the ENP as:

> an Accident and Emergency nurse who has a sound nursing practice in all aspects of Accident and Emergency nursing, with formal post-basic education in holistic assessment, physical diagnosis, in prescription of treatment and in the promotion of health.

This definition clarifies neither 'sound nursing practice' nor the level of the post-basic education. The RCN Ruling Council (Royal College of Nursing 1996) agreed that a nurse practitioner can be identified as a nurse who:

- has undertaken a specific course of study of at least first-degree (honours) level;
- makes professionally autonomous decisions for which he or she has sole responsibility;
- receives patients with undifferentiated and undiagnosed problems, and makes an assessment of their health-care needs based on highly developed nursing knowledge and skills not usually exercised by nurses, such as physical examination;
- screens patients for disease risk factors and early signs of illness;
- develops with the patient an ongoing nursing care plan for health, with an emphasis on preventive measures;
- provides counselling and health education;
- has the authority to admit or discharge patients from his or her own caseload and refer them to other health-care providers as appropriate.

This definition, however, stems from a predominantly primary care focus, for example 'develops with the patient an ongoing nursing care plan for health, with an emphasis on preventive measures', and may have reduced applicability within the emergency care setting. Read and George's (1994) definition that 'nurse practitioners are authorised to treat patients, either as an alternative to being seen by a doctor, or in the absence of a doctor at the site' is more inclusive; however, it does not explicitly refer to the educational preparation required for the role. For the purposes of this book, the ENP is defined as:

> a nurse working within an acute, emergency care setting who has undertaken a specific course of study to enable him or her to make professionally autonomous decisions for which he or she has sole responsibility, and who can assess, treat, refer and discharge patients without recourse to a medical practitioner.

Clinical activities of ENPs

Hicks and Hennessy (1998) suggest that the role of the nurse practitioner should include advanced clinical and psychosocial skills to cover patient assessment, care planning, referral and clinical decision-making. In addition, they argue, a high level of communication skill is essential in order for the nurse practitioner to function effectively within the multidisciplinary team as well as in an enhanced clinical role. The clinical activities that ENPs undertake can vary considerably and, at the risk of being prescriptive, may include assessing and managing minor lacerations, burns, soft tissue injuries, throat and other relatively minor infections, suturing wounds, the prescription of analgesia and antibiotics, the management of limb fractures and so on (Dolan & Dale 1997, Dolan et al 1997).

There are no nationally agreed guidelines for practice, the minimum educational attainment of nurse practitioners or even standards at which such advanced practice should be undertaken (Walsh 1997, UKCC 1998). The South East Thames Regional Health Authority (1994) has recommended 'the employment of a properly trained nurse specialist [or practitioner] to treat the patient according to protocols which can be audited'. Fawcett-Henesy (1991) considered that there were seven characteristics of nurse practitioner practice:

1. direct access for patients;
2. a choice for patients (nurse practitioner versus doctor);
3. diagnostic and prescribing skills;
4. authority for referral;
5. personal attention during consultation;
6. adequate time for consultation;
7. counselling and health education.

The characteristics described by Fawcett-Henesy allow for the development of the role, although 'counselling' in its narrow sense is probably beyond the scope of most nurse practitioners' practice. Walsh (1989), however, asks whether 'nurse practitioner' is a valid concept or whether it is just the case of nurses wanting to 'play' at being doctors. Ford and Walsh (1994) criticize Howie (1992) for introducing a scheme in which the nurse practitioner was only employed when he or she was available and the doctor was not. They believe that this provides clear evidence of the nurse working as a doctor substitute rather than as a nurse practitioner.

James and Pyrgos (1989) looked at the theoretical management of walking wounded patients by four experienced A&E sisters who had worked in A&E departments for more than five years. Their decisions were compared with those made by post-fellowship registrars or full-time clinical assistants. Four hundred patients, who did not have head, eye, chest or abdominal complaints, other than superficial wounds, took part in the study. Of the total of 400 patients seen, 3 refused to take part in the trial. Of the remaining 397 patients, 65 were referred directly to the doctor. The nursing staff thus saw and assessed 332 patients.

The patients saw the nurse first and were examined. The nurse recorded the diagnosis and treatment, as well as whether an X-ray would be requested. The patients were then returned to their original position in the queue to see the doctor; this was to allow any potential saving in time to be assessed. The doctors did not know any details of the nurses' decisions before they saw the patient.

Out of the 397 patients in the study seen by the nurses, only 3% (12) were 'mismanaged'. Both the doctor and the nurse felt that 150 of the patients required an X-ray. Twenty-two patients would have been X-rayed by the nurse only, but as they were *not* X-rayed, it is impossible to say for certain whether any of these patients had a missed fracture, although the study does point out that none of these patients had returned within 1 month with further problems arising from the injury. Eighteen patients were, on the other hand, X-rayed by the doctor and not by the nurses: in 4 of these 18, a fracture was revealed on X-ray.

Out of the 142 patients for whom both the doctor and the nurse agreed that an X-ray was not required, the doctor and nurse agreed on the diagnosis in 137 cases, although 5 of these would have received unsatisfactory treatment, according to local practice, had the nurses treated them. Of the 5 cases for which differing diagnoses were made, 1 would have received the same treatment anyway, and 2 more would have received satisfactory treatment. Two would have received unsatisfactory care. Looking at the 12 'mismanaged cases', 4 were missed fractures, 1 was a missed ganglion on a flexor tendon, and the other 7 all related to either failing to prescribe drugs (5) or prescribing drugs to which the patient had an allergy (2). As the nurses had no specific training for the role, and if better patient selection criteria were used, it would be reasonable to assume that the already low percentage of 'mismanaged cases' would be lowered still further.

The authors of this study note that the nurses' examination technique relied more on experience and intuition than on method. This paper demonstrates that experienced A&E nurses, with no specific nurse practitioner training, can perform well in treating most patients when compared with experienced A&E middle-grade doctors. The study also demonstrated a theoretical saving of 11 minutes waiting time per patient if they saw a nurse rather than a doctor: 17 minutes waiting compared with 28. Of the 332 patients seen by the nurses, 311 (94%) stated that they would have been happy to be treated by a suitably trained nurse for an appropriate condition. This article did not consider the consultation behaviour of the nurses, focusing exclusively on a biomedical model of patient management. It is worth stressing, nevertheless, that nursing assessment is different from medical history-taking as it places more emphasis on psychosocial dimensions of care. However, the authors note that the nurses performed well in terms of patient outcome.

A more recent study by Meek et al (1998) showed that nurse practitioners performed significantly better than inexperienced junior doctors when requesting and interpreting X-rays. Nurse practitioners in 13 A&E departments or MIUs were shown 20 X-rays of limbs, with a brief history and examination findings, and asked to record their interpretations. A total score for each participant was calculated by comparing the answers against agreed responses. Fifty-eight nurse practitioners, 43 experienced senior house officers (SHOs), that is, those in their sixth month working in A&E, and 41 inexperienced SHOs, those in their first month in A&E, were tested.

The nurse practitioners as a whole performed significantly better than the inexperienced SHO group, and while the experienced SHO group performed better than the nurse practitioners, the difference was not significant. The researchers' recommendation of expanding the ENP role to include X-ray interpretation appears to be safe, providing that the safeguards applied to SHO interpretation are also used for ENPs. Strikingly, the nurse practitioners in this study performed only marginally less well than the experienced SHOs in interpreting X-rays, even though they had no formal training in doing so. Indeed, no information is provided by Meek et al (1998) about the amount and type of training that those working as nurse practitioners had received.

There appears to be an implicit assumption in many such studies that ENPs perform well despite being nurses who have not had the same training opportunities as their medical colleagues. As Prescott et al (1981) have noted, 'even though a large number of studies indicate that nurse practitioners outperformed physicians in certain areas that were evaluated, their superior performance is seldom recognised' (p 223). Instead, a commonly drawn conclusion is that there are no differences between nurse practitioners' and doctors' performances in those areas (Prescott & Driscoll 1979). It also presumes that physician practice is generally an adequate and acceptable standard against which to evaluate nurse practitioner practice. Prescott and Driscoll (1980) argue that it is reasonable to suspect that there would be a significant difference (favouring nurses) if the basis of the comparison were patient teaching, consultation, counselling or other activities related to the supportive function of the care role. While the proposed research is not a comparative study, it may be possible to draw some conclusions based on the final results of the consultation analysis.

Comparative studies of nurse practitioners and doctors show that nurse practitioners are as effective as doctors when assessing, diagnosing and treating patients with minor injuries and illnesses. This suggests that the clinical activities of ENPs as outlined above are practised without compromising patient safety. It would also be true to suggest that the work of Meek et al (1998) appears to legitimize what nurses had undertaken surreptitiously for a number of years, and for which they are gaining increasing recognition. This may in part relate to the more equitable consultation that the patients receive. In the next section, a range of consultation studies will be considered, leading to the development of questions that could be investigated empirically.

Consultation studies

Consultation and communication studies appeared to gain legitimacy in the 1960s and 70s as 'scientific' approaches were developed to measure interactions between doctors and patients. A number of studies refer the 'need' for scientific inquiry or attempts at quantification (for example, Korsch et al 1968, Freeman et al 1971). Roter (1989) notes that the evolution of methodological and technological sophistication has made the observation and analysis of the medical visit easier over the years.

While there are a substantial number of doctor–patient consultation studies (Pendleton 1983, Beisecker & Beisecker 1990, Arborelius & Bremberg 1992, Butler et al 1992, Baker 1996), there is little published research examining nurse–patient communication in the A&E department. A small study by Wood (1979), using structured observation, supports the common finding that nurses' interaction with patients is brief, predominantly task centred and concerned with physical care. Nurses appeared to restrict their contact with patients to those interactions which were necessary for the patients' progress through the department. Wood used only a small sample of 20 patients with minor injuries, using a precoded structured checklist to classify the types of interaction that occurred. No contextual detail was provided, making it difficult to explain the reasons for the limited communication observed.

Another more recent study by Byrne and Heyman (1997), based on a PhD study undertaken by Byrne (1992), used a symbolic interactionist perspective to understand nurses' communication in A&E. This approach aims to understand the social group studied by exploring the relationship between social structure and the meanings by which individuals interpret and create their social world. The research involved structured interviews with patients to identify the sources of anxiety for patients in A&E, in-depth interviews with nurses in two A&E departments to explore their perceptions of their work and patients, and an observational study examining the nature of nurse–patient communication in A&E. Whereas this paper only considers the interviews with nurses, the authors state that the observations support the descriptions of nursing actions reported at interview. This study considered the work of A&E nurses rather than nurse practitioners, and participants in the study made it abundantly clear that minor illness and injuries care, the bread-and-butter work of ENPs, did not interest them. It was undertaken at a time when ENPs were uncommon, and the proposed research may, it is hoped, help to fill this gap in the literature.

In a study not dissimilar to the one proposed, Johnson (1993) focused on nurse practitioner–patient conversations in a primary care setting. Transcripts from 24 audiotaped nurse practitioner–patient conversations and three nurse practitioner research interviews, as well as 100 hours of field notes from observations, were analysed using a combination of discourse and ethnographic analysis. This study took place at a medical clinic in the outpatient department. The three nurse practitioners who took part were women with 2–15 years experience. The selection criteria for patients participating in the study were that they were women and spoke English. The 22 patients were white, between the ages of 31 and 86 (mean age = 61) and predominantly from middle to lower socio-economic groups. While Johnson (1993) justifies her exclusion of male patients on the grounds that she was interested in woman-to-woman talk, this nonetheless weakens the study as it cannot be ascertained whether men and women receive different consultation approaches from the nurse practitioners.

Using discourse analysis, Johnson (1993) posits that a pattern was evident for a negotiable agenda that was established through the use of open-ended questions, eliciting information from the patient, conducting the physical examination and developing a plan of care. In this way, she believes, the 'voice' of nursing in primary care practice is revealed. In a response to Johnson's paper, Brykczynski (1993, p 159) agrees that:

> these hybrid nurses (nurse practitioners) who incorpo-
> rate medical components into the nursing perspective
> can be understood as bicultural and bilingual. They are
> fluent in the voice of medicine and the voice of patients
> (the lifeworld).

One innovation outside nursing, but perhaps with useful lessons for practice, was undertaken by Dale et al (1991). GPs were introduced into an A&E department with the aim of delivering care to patients who presented with primary care needs. It was found that they requested fewer diagnostic tests, such as X-rays, laid a greater emphasis on listening, and were more flexible in their use of time than were their A&E SHO colleagues. This was without any raised incidence of patient dissatisfaction or evidence of undertreatment. One interesting finding from this study for the emerging nurse practitioner may, however, arise from the fact that very few consultations with either GPs or casualty officers included a discussion of the patient's lifestyle, such as issues of smoking, diet or exercise. It would be important to establish whether nurse practitioner consultations address these issues.

Estimates as high as 40% have been made of patients attending inner-city A&E departments with primary health-care problems (Dale 1992). A common response to this is that nurse practitioners may have a place in inner-city departments for dealing with patients with minor illnesses that could be managed in a GP's surgery, but not in more rural locations with a better uptake of community facilities. However, Dolan and Dale (1997) found that patients attending two MIUs had conditions remarkably similar to those which would be expected in a larger A&E department. Both of these units were in rural environments with reasonably high-quality primary care services.

Salisbury and Tettersell (1988) propose that the nurse practitioner may well provide an extra service rather than acting as a doctor substitute. It is worth briefly exploring the implicit assumption behind this statement. Doctors train with an illness perspective emphasizing physical disease and treatment, whereas nurse training places a greater emphasis on practical teaching and advice. Both are necessary, and are complementary in providing comprehensive health-care facilities in any setting.

There is, however, an unstated assumption that health-care services as provided by physicians are adequate in every respect except quantity (Diers & Molde 1979). The relative status in society of doctors and nurses may also affect the consultation relationship (Poulton 1996). Evidence appears to suggest that patients can talk more easily with nurses, whereas they fear that questioning the doctor too much might be wasteful of his or her time (Stilwell 1985). Salisbury and Tettersell (1988) found that nurse practitioner–patient consultations were longer than doctor–patient consultations; thus, more time could be spent in identifying problems, exploring potential solutions and evaluating outcomes. Prescott & Driscoll (1980), however, suggest that whereas more time per patient might be a sign of a high quality of care, one could also argue that the greater time represents reduced efficiency, insecurity or incompetence on the part of the practitioner.

Dolan et al (1997) have also suggested that the longer consultation times of nurse practitioners may make them less economically viable in a resource-stretched NHS as they see fewer cases, leading to a relatively high cost per patient episode. Dolan et al (1997), however, fail to acknowledge that nurse practitioner consultation times usually include nursing time, whereas the consultation times of junior doctors do not. This means that while a junior doctor will examine and diagnose, for example, a sprained ankle, he or she will then usually ask the nurse to treat the condition while the doctor sees another patient or writes up the case notes. In practice, a nurse practitioner will also treat the patient's condition, which adds to the length of the consultation but leads to more holistic care, being, it is suggested, more satisfying for the patient.

A constant comparison with doctors' practice, while necessary in terms of safety and cost-effectiveness for equitable provision, perhaps disguises some of the value of skilled nursing. Instead of basing practice on task performance, Stilwell (1991) identified five areas of work for which the nurse practitioner could take responsibility:

1. acting as an alternative consultant for the patient;
2. detecting serious disease by physical examination;
3. managing minor and chronic ailments and injuries;
4. providing health education;
5. counselling.

Doctors may well argue that they too can provide these services. Bliss (1976) supports this and suggests that nurse practitioner development is often argued on two questionable assumptions: first, that doctors will not or cannot provide health maintenance and care; and second, that cure and care are mutually exclusive. Bliss proposes instead that a continuum exists along which medicine and nursing oscillate, and that by combining both cure and care in the same health-care provider, both process and outcome measures may be maximized.

All the studies described above suggest that patients found seeing a nurse practitioner to be acceptable, often viewing it as an improvement in the service. Patients also appeared to appreciate the more relaxed and equal style of consultation offered by the nurse practitioner. Stanford (1987), however, has described areas such as nurse practitioner–patient consultations as a 'neglected' area for research. A criticism of much research into nurse–patient communication, where it has been undertaken, is that the contribution of the patient is ignored (Jarrett & Payne 1995). As patient satisfaction is one objective of care, and, along with recovery from illness or the amelioration of the presenting problem, also an outcome of care (Baker 1990), it would seem appropriate that any study into nurse practitioner–patient consultations should incorporate patients' views. In addition, a consideration of how the nurse also viewed the consultation with the patient seems important, as the expectations for each party may be different, which could affect the establishment of the nurse–patient relationship.

Conclusion

This chapter has outlined the development of the nurse practitioner role with particular reference to ENPs who practise in A&E and MIUs. The problems associated with definition, and with studies of the clinical activities of ENPs, have also been considered, before outlining a range of studies into nurse practitioner–patient consultations. The relative lack of these, especially studies that incorporate patients' views, is a feature of the literature.

This leads to the development of a number of questions about nurse practitioner–patient consultation that could be addressed by empirical investigation. These questions and their methodological implications will be addressed in the next chapter.

Chapter 3
Methodological discussion

This chapter will critically examine a range of methodological issues relating to undertaking this pilot study. It will identify the aims and objectives of the research, as well as the research questions that will be investigated in the study. A number of methodological issues, for example access, ethical issues and sampling, will be explored. In addition, the range of research instruments used will be outlined and their use justified.

This pilot study aims:

- To analyse the process and content of nurse practitioner consultations and appraise patient satisfaction in A&E departments.

Its objectives are:

- To test a research tool to describe the nurse practitioner consultation process and content in an A&E department.
- To test a research tool to describe the nurse practitioner's perceptions of the consultation.
- To test a research tool to assess patient satisfaction with nurse practitioner consultations.
- To test a research tool to audit the case notes of nurse practitioner consultations.

Research questions

The following are the questions to be asked by the research:

- What are the process and content of ENP consultations in A&E departments and MIUs?

- How do ENP and patient perceptions about the consultation process compare in A&E departments and MIUs in terms of satisfaction?
- How does the nurse practitioner's documentation of the consultation compare with a structured analysis of the consultation's process and content?

In seeking to address these aims, objectives and research questions in this pilot study, a number of methodological issues should be considered before examining the fitness for purpose of the research instruments themselves. These methodological issues are considered in the next section.

Methodological issues

Methodological issues relate to the theoretical and practical issues associated with undertaking research. Cohen and Manion (1994, p 39) describe the aim of methodology as 'to help us to understand, in the broadest possible terms, not the products of scientific enquiry but the process itself'. They differentiate this from methods, which they define as 'that range of approaches used in educational research to gather data which are to be used as a basis for inference and interpretation, for explanation and prediction' (Cohen & Manion 1994, p 38). This section will consider the methodology of the study, including some of these processes and approaches relating to methods.

Access

The initial problem at the outset of most research is that of gaining access to the field of study (Wolcott 1995). Knowing who has the power to open up or block off access, or who consider themselves or are considered by others to have the authority to grant or refuse access, is a critically important aspect of field research (Hammersley & Atkinson 1995). Those who exercise control over physical access and information are termed 'gatekeepers' and play a significant role in research (Burgess 1990). The gatekeepers in this pilot study were the senior ENP and his ENP colleagues, the Director of Nursing, the A&E Nurse Manager and the local ethics committee.

Hammersley and Atkinson (1995) have noted that the discovery of obstacles to access, and perhaps of an effective means of overcoming them, provides insights into the social organization of the setting. Burgess (1984, p 51) recommends that 'access should not merely be negotiated with those who occupy the highest position in a social situation but with different individuals so as to avoid misunderstanding'. Researchers frequently rely upon personal contacts to find sponsors; indeed, research settings are often selected, and access facilitated, because researchers have some prior experience of, or contact with, the group or institution (Foster 1996). In this instance, the senior ENP acted as a sponsor, facilitating meetings with other ENP staff and the Director of Nursing. His credibility was critical in garnering support from among the staff for this study.

Ethical issues

The ethics of research in nursing must be consistent with the ethics of nursing practice (National Institute for Nursing 1993, Royal College of Nursing 1998). All research conducted within the auspices of the NHS and involving human participants or personal information relating to them requires the approval of the local ethics committee. Permission must be granted by the committee before research can begin. For the pilot study, a standard form was completed and 34 copies of the ethics approval form submitted to the committee secretariat.

Ethics committees are generally made up of doctors, lay people and usually, but not always, nurses. They are particularly concerned with issues such as informed consent, confidentiality and anonymity, as well as with preventing the exploitation of and harm to participants. In the current study, written consent (Appendix I) was required from all respondents, who were also given an explanatory letter and an information sheet (Appendix II) and advised that they could withdraw from the study at any time without it affecting their treatment in any way. In the past, many researchers were reluctant to provide such information to participants because they felt that to do so might influence the outcome of the research. Benton and Cormack (1996) argue that such a stance is no longer defensible, and any research seeking to hide information from a participant will not be given approval by the ethics committee.

Confidentiality and anonymity are frequently seen as being synonymous in research, but they are subtly different. While information may be given in confidence, it may not be possible for it to remain anonymous. In this study, there were only four nurse practitioners, and as each obviously knew the others, it was not possible to ensure that the identities of each respondent would be unknown to the rest, resulting in what Rauch (cited in McKenna 1994) calls 'quasi-anonymity', implying that while the respondents might be known to one another, their judgements and opinions could remain strictly anonymous. As a result, information given in confidence could not be anonymous beyond the fact that the individual identity of the respondent could be guessed at with a 1 in 3 chance of being right, assuming that the person guessing was also one of the sample group.

For the patients, once the study's information entered the public domain – for example if this dissertation were deposited in a university library, or its content published in journal articles – it would technically be no longer confidential. Anonymity can, however, be assured as the information gleaned could not reasonably be expected to identify individual patients. For the reasons outlined above, nurse practitioner anonymity could not be guaranteed, but the practitioners had given their informed consent to take part in the study and did not mind that they were potentially identifiable. This does not, however, absolve the researcher from aspiring to maintain both confidentiality and anonymity, so a coded number to identify the individual respondents, known only to the researcher, was given to the ENPs and patients involved in the study.

Assurances regarding the confidentiality of patient data were also provided in the information sheet given to prospective patient participants, who were advised that the audiotapes would be stored under lock and key and, once the study was completed, would be destroyed rather being taped over in other research projects. The transcripts of the nurse practitioner consultations would also be destroyed, and the floppy disk holding this information stored with the audiotapes and in due course erased. The purpose of this was further to reduce the risk of breaches of patient confidentiality. In addition, the identity of ENP respondents and the hospital would not be revealed in this dissertation. While a copy of the dissertation would, as promised, be sent to the staff at the pilot site concerned, it is recommended good practice not to reveal information that could breach these confidences, such as identifying the hospital involved.

Preventing exploitation and harm to respondents has echoes of Florence Nightingale's dictum that 'First, the hospital should do the patient no harm'. Being honest with patients and assuring them that they can withdraw at any time from the study without compromising the care they received was critical. While stressing to patients that they would not directly benefit from the research, it was highlighted that their support of the study would provide greater insights and understanding into the role and activities of the ENP. This meant that no patients were under any illusion that they would receive preferential or different treatment as a result of taking part in the study. The need to avoid as far as possible exploiting the goodwill of the ENPs themselves was also critically important. Their names were not used in the study, and as noted above, it was agreed that feedback in the form of a copy of the dissertation would be provided. Opportunities were also created to provide intermediate feedback to the ENP respondents in the form of informally discussing with them their consultation experience.

Identifying the research strategy

Each research strategy has particular advantages and disadvantages, depending, according to Yin (1994), on three conditions:

1. the type of research question;
2. how much control an investigator has over actual behavioural events;
3. the focus on contemporary as opposed to historical phenomena.

A fourth condition, I would suggest, would include the background, values, belief system and research paradigm of the investigator.

The research strategy used for this pilot was a case study. In general, case studies are preferred when the investigator has little control over events, and when the focus is on a contemporary phenomenon within some real-life context (Yin 1994). A case – the focus of the study – is an individual informant or participant engaged in a sequence of activities over a period of time, in this instance as a nurse practitioner or patient involved in the consultation. Mitchell (1983) believes that it is not the content of the case study that is important, but the use to which the data are put to support any theoretical conclusions. Hammersley and Atkinson (1995) view a case as being an object of study that is distinct from the study setting because it is examined from one rather than multiple theoretical angles.

In general, the unit of analysis adopted here is the consultation content and process of nurse practitioners and patients. A small number of cases are studied because the focus is on discovery rather than simple enumeration; however, a range of strategies to uncover the consultation content and process is adopted.

Sampling

In this study, a range of exclusion criteria were established:

- patients requiring immediate or urgent care, for example because of bleeding, pain or distress;
- patients under 18 years of age;
- those unable to give informed consent;
- those who acknowledged themselves to be functionally illiterate or who were unable to comprehend and complete the post-consultation questionnaire.

As there was a large Turkish and Kurdish community in the catchment area of the hospital, an interpreter/advocate was on hand to translate for members of this community as appropriate. In the event, her expertise was sought only once, and it was quickly established that the potential respondent had learning difficulties and would thus have been unable to provide informed consent. The person concerned was then excluded from the study.

The sampling approach is purposive, a sample being built up that enables the researcher to meet the specific needs of the project; this is an approach commonly used within case studies (Yin 1994). The selection strategy was of a non-probability type, in which there is no means of estimating the probability of units (cases) being selected (Burgess 1984). An opportunistic sample, based on those patients who happened to meet the inclusion criteria and who presented to the primary care/minor injuries unit (PC/MIU) was included in the study. While there is no reason to believe that those included in the study were representative of the population, the fact that the unit was open from 8 am to 8 pm, and that the researcher was available for these opening times, means that a good cross-section of the patients presenting to the unit were recruited. The corollary, therefore, is that there is no evidence to suggest that the sample is not representative of the population.

The study was set in the PC/MIU of an A&E department in the South of England. Nurses and patients were selected from this setting. The A&E department, including the PC/MIU, sees approximately 50 000 new patients per annum. As noted in the literature review in Chapter 2, ENPs in the unit see patients with a range of minor illness and injuries, including, for example, lacerations, limb fractures and chest infections.

Quantitative and qualitative research

The quantitative world is characterized as being hypothetico-deductive, particularistic, objective and outcome oriented, its researchers being seen as logical positivists. In contrast, the qualitative world view is characterized as social anthropological, inductive, holistic, subjective and process oriented (Roter & Frankel 1992), its researchers being non-positivists, such as phenomenologists, constructivists and ethnomethodologists. The controversy over the relative values of the qualitative and quantitative approaches to nursing research for understanding human behaviour has been a source of growing debate among nursing scholars (Schultz 1992, Ford-Gilboe et al 1995, Shih 1998).

Shih (1998) suggests the discipline of nursing needs methodological strategies that will enhance nurse researchers' efforts to describe and conceptualize the multifaceted complexity of the human response to illness and various health-care situations. In recognition of this need, there is a growing emphasis on combining qualitative and quantitative methods in a single study (Goodwin & Goodwin 1984, Abbott & Sapsford 1998). However, it is worth stressing that the combination of qualitative and quantitative methods does not necessarily lead to triangulation. Triangulation is a procedure used to establish the fact that the criterion of validity has been met. It can, but does not necessarily, include the use of multiple data sources, multiple methods and so on. The key point is that one is examining a single social phenomenon from more than a single vantage point. In the case of this pilot study, a major strength of case study data collection is the opportunity to use many different sources of evidence.

Yin (1994) notes that the most important advantage present by using multiple sources of evidence is the development of converging lines of inquiry, which is a process of triangulation. Thus, any finding or conclusion is likely to be much more convincing and accurate if it is based on several different sources of information following a corroboratory mode. This study sought that sort of corroboration.

Validity and reliability

Whilst Eisner (1991) has argued that validity and reliability are not useful, they are still perceived to be important dimensions of the rigour of research studies. LeCompte and Goetz (1982, p 31) argue that 'the value of scientific research is partially dependent on the ability of individual researchers to demonstrate the credibility of their findings. Regardless of the discipline of the methods used for data collection and analysis', they add, 'all scientific ways of knowing strive for authentic results'.

External reliability addresses the issue of whether independent research would discover the same phenomena or generate the same constructs in the same or similar settings. It is regarded as being less important in case studies as one is not looking for generalizability of the findings (Schofield 1993). Internal reliability refers to the degree to which other researchers, given a set of previously generated constructs, would match them with data in the same way as did the original researcher. Because of factors such as the uniqueness or complexity of phenomena, qualitative research, including this study, may approach rather than attain external reliability (Bowling 1997). However, whereas reliability is concerned with the replicability of scientific findings, validity is concerned with their accuracy. It is hoped that the transparency of use of the research instruments in this study will enhance confidence in the pilot. The next section will describe the research instruments that will be used.

Research instruments

Street (1992) argues that researchers should consider utilizing multiple measures of communication within the same study. For example, she suggests, one research strategy would be to use measures garnered from both observers and participants. Such a tactic provides data on the patient's perspective as well as generating an independent assessment of the communicative events of the consultation. In this study, a range of instruments have been piloted. The consultation between the patient and the ENP was recorded, the patient was asked to complete a Medical Interview Satisfaction Scale (MISS; Appendix III), the ENP was asked to complete a post-consultation question-naire (Appendix IV), and finally an audit of the clinical content of the nurse practitioner case notes (Appendix V) was undertaken. This section will outline the use and theoretical issues associated with each of these instruments.

Audiotaping nurse practitioner–patient consultations

The use of audiotape recordings allows for an analysis of both linguistic and paralinguistic cues ('ums' and 'aahs') but excludes kinesic information, such as gestures, facial expression and body relationship. Direct observation and videotape recordings are the only observational strategies that allow for the study of the linguistic, paralinguistic and kinesic transfer of information. To reduce intrusiveness and enhance patient comfort and confiden-tiality, the nurse practitioner wore a microphone whose signal was picked up on a radio receiver connected to a tape-recorder, so that the researcher did not have to be present with the patient and nurse practitioner during the consultation. The reason for this was to reduce the observer effect (Foster 1996), which could have unduly influenced both the patient's and nurse practitioner's consultation process and content.

The audiotapes were analysed using the Multi-dimensional Interaction Analysis (MDIA) system, which was designed by two social scientists and two doctors to study interactions between doctors and their elderly patients (Greene et al 1987, Adelman et al 1991). The MDIA allows the researcher studying medical interac-tions to capture the context, content and meaning of the interactions with a method that allows for a fairly streamlined coding of the sessions from the audiotapes. Combining features of the process analysis approach and micro-analytic approach, the MDIA is founded on the recognition that nurse–patient interactions are story-telling sessions during which the patient narrates that which happened, and the nurse, ideally, makes narrative sense of that which is told (Charon et al 1994).

The MDIA conceptualizes the nurse practitioner–patient inter-view as two simultaneous interviews: the nurse interviewing the patient, and the patient interviewing the nurse. Both nurse and patient raise issues or topics in these interviews. Both interviews are conducted in certain ways; that is, there are the interviewing behaviours or processes of both participants to be recorded and assessed. An interview is a mutual enterprise in which speakers address one another by name or title, for example 'nurse', turns are taken, dominance may occur, emotion may be expressed, laughter may be shared, and decisions may be made mutually or unilaterally. Both participants in the interview can be evaluated for their demonstration of such global characteristics as assertiveness or respectfulness. Finally, the consultation itself can be globally characterized using such descriptors as 'warm', 'trusting' or 'superfi-cial'. The MDIA addresses all these aspects of the patient's visit. In this study, piloting sought to establish whether the MDIA would be sufficiently sensitive to use in the larger-scale study that would then follow.

Medical Interview Satisfaction Scale

The MISS is an internally consistent, easily administered measure of three aspects of patient satisfaction: cognitive, affective and behav-ioural (Appendix III). The scale yields a broader distribution of scores than has been reported for other similar scales. The MISS measures satisfaction with a particular interview as distinct from general attitudes towards doctors or health-care services. Because items in the MISS refer directly to a specific patient–provider interaction, it is likely to be more sensitive to actual differences in care than are measures of general attitudes (Wolfe et al 1978).

Correlations of the scale with demographic variables are low or non-significant, which suggests that these factors do not seriously contaminate responses. Other evidence (Stiles et al 1978) suggests that the cognitive and affective subscales are significantly correlated with measures of clinically relevant patient and physician behaviours. The MISS was administered as a questionnaire to patients following their consultation with the nurse practitioner. It was modified to incorporate the term 'nurse practitioner' rather than 'doctor', but otherwise no changes were made. The MISS incorporates a 5-point Likert scale to rate the patient's perceived significance of the item (Foddy 1994).

Post-consultation nurse practitioner questionnaire

This was given to the ENPs immediately following their consultation with the patient. In designing the questionnaire, the questions asked of the ENPs were tailored around the research questions for the study (Appendix IV). The first part asked details about the patient, such as gender, age/date of birth, main symptoms present and so on, in order to allow the cross-tabulation of datasets. A 5-point Likert scale in the second half of the questionnaire asked the nurse practitioners how they felt about the consultation. In many respects, this questionnaire mimicked the MISS, but it also asked open-ended questions about whether there were any problems with consultations and whether there was anyone else, other than the patient, present. A further open-ended question at the end of the questionnaire provided the ENP with the opportunity to make any further comments about the consultation in question. The questionnaire was ordered in this way, as recommended by Moser and Kalton (1971), to enable the respondent to answer straightforward, simple questions first before being asked more challenging ones.

Audit of case notes

Although notoriously incomplete and unstandardized, case note review is often the primary source of information in formal procedures of evaluating care (Donabedian 1968, Heartfield 1996). Most importantly, case notes do not ordinarily contain information about either the nursing care provided or the variables that might be considered measures of the effect of nursing, such as psychosocial concerns and domestic arrangements. At best, case notes contain only indirect measures of the art of care. Although nurse practitioners may spend a significant amount of time discussing health-promotion issues with the patient, this may be recorded simply as 'health advice given', thus rendering almost invisible one of the most crucial elements of the nurse practitioner's role: to see patients in the context of their own lifestyles, and to deliver care and advice accordingly.

The case note recording of existing nurse practitioner practice tends to favour the medical model approach (Appendix V). This, however, appears to be at odds with the value-added approach that nurse practitioners bring to their role, that is, their use of both nursing and medical knowledge to create a hybrid knowledge that is more holistic in nature and comprehensive in delivery. The under-recognition of the nursing dimensions of care in case notes serves to illegitimize nursing practice, placing it in a subordinate position to medical skills, which tend to be the key area of practice that is recognized in recording the nurse practitioner's encounter with the patient. Heartfield (1996) goes further and argues that the dominant power of institutional, scientific and medical knowledge and processes is clearly evident in the way in which nursing is mediated through the patient case note.

In this study, a tool devised by Dale et al (1991) was used to audit the case notes of the nurse practitioners. This was originally devised in order to audit the clinical content of the case notes of GPs working as primary care physicians in the A&E department at King's College Hospital, London. The training of GPs, indeed all postgraduate medical training with the possible exception of psychiatry, places great emphasis on the psychosocial context of a patient's illness as well as identifying the traditional biophysical dimensions of his or her malaise. This, it is intended, should lead to a more holistic approach to the care of patients, and in many respects reflects the imbuing philosophy underlying nurse practitioner practice, which is to see the patient as a complex social entity rather than a vessel for disease or injury.

Lynaugh and Bates (1973) put it more bluntly when describing the results of the differing medical and nursing perspectives. They argue that the physician tends to emphasize structure, whether normal or diseased, whereas the nurse is more concerned with function. This translates to a disease orientation for physicians and a person orientation for nurses. In fairness, they may not have had British GPs in mind when they made their comments, as many do not work in the hospital setting for the very reason that they eschew this reductionist biomedical paradigm favoured by some of their hospital-based medical colleagues.

The case note audit tool used in this study, although designed for GPs, would, it was hoped, be sensitive enough to illustrate the dimensions of nurse practitioner consultation recording without making invisible the nursing domains of practice.

Justifying the use of these research instruments

This pilot study is complex because a range of research instruments are being used to address the research questions. Instead of simply analysing nurse practitioner–patient consultations by audiotaping them, the study sought to understand the whole process from both a patient and a nurse perspective. It is important, therefore, to justify the use of these individual research tools in order explain why they, rather than perhaps other approaches, were considered to be best suited to answer the research questions being addressed.

The Multi-dimensional Interaction Analysis tool

The MDIA is a well-validated research tool that has been used in a number of other studies (for example, Henbest & Stewart 1990). In identifying the story that the patient has to tell, and the nurse's exploration and understanding of that narrative, it is believed that the MDIA will allow the explication of this important dimension of nursing practice to be uncovered. Other analytic tools, such as those used by Chambers (1996, 1998), rely simply on a post-consultation questionnaire (posted to respondents some time after their visit to a GP); and sociolinguistic studies, for example those by Skopek (1979) and Cassell et al (1977), are concerned with language, attempting to categorize each utterance into types such as 'acoustic', 'phonological', 'syntactic' and 'lexical'. Pendleton (1983) notes that sociolinguistic studies are extremely expensive and time-consuming to analyse, as well as being relatively unsophisticated in terms of making the interaction genuinely interactional.

Studies of non-verbal behaviour in the consultation were not possible because the mechanism for capturing data was audio- rather than videotaping. This approach was used by Byrne and Heath (1980), who studied non-verbal behaviour in relation to verbal exchanges and suggested that non-verbal behaviour can aid or hinder communication, sometimes even preventing it. Although this has become a widely quoted paper, it is not the intention of this research to explore this matter; instead, the MDIA will be used to consider both the story-telling and narrative of the nurse and patient's experience.

The Medical Interview Satisfaction Scale

The MISS, as designed by Wolfe et al (1978), is also a validated tool that has been used in numerous settings. In their search of patient satisfaction studies since the 1960s, these authors found only two scales that measured the patient's perception of an initial health-care encounter directly and systematically (Vuori et al 1972, Risser 1975). There were, however, problems with each in terms of reliability and validity.

Since then, Baker (1996) has developed a Consultation Satisfaction Scale comprising 18 questions in four scales concerned with general satisfaction, professional care, depth of relationship and perceived time. This has been shown to have satisfactory levels of internal consistency, test–retest reliability and validity. The difficulty with it for the purposes of this study is that while it is, as Baker (1996, p 603) argues, 'a robust measure to determine the characteristics of patients, GPs and their practices that influence patient satisfaction with consultations in general practice', it seeks to understand the patients' opinions of the organization of practices, rather than, as highlighted by the MISS, the consultation process and content itself. It is because the MISS focuses on the patient's perspective of the consultation rather than the organization of care or the consultation environment that it was used for this study.

The post-consultation nurse practitioner questionnaire

As Pendleton (1983) notes, research into complex phenomena is inevitably fragmented since no individual study can hope to be exhaustive. Attempts can be made, however, to be as comprehensive as possible in order to get differing dimensions of practice that serve to buttress one another in terms of their trustworthiness (Guba 1981). For this reason, the ENPs in the study were invited to complete a post-consultation questionnaire. As no similar questionnaire could be found in the literature, it was necessary to design one, which, it was hoped, would be sensitive enough to detect information on the ease of the consultation for the ENP concerned. As well as patient data, a Likert scale and open-ended questions were used. It was estimated that it would take respondents 3–5 minutes to complete.

Audit of clinical content of nurse practitioner records

As noted previously, GP practice tends to take a psychosocial as well as a biophysical perspective on patient care. For this reason, it was hoped that this tool would be sensitive enough to capture such information from the case note recordings of the ENPs. Other audit tools, such as that used by Dale and Dolan (1996), have focused on the following details documented in the case notes: presenting problem, time and date of attendance, postcode of residence, age, sex, diagnosis and referral/discharge. While this study sought to establish whether patients used MIUs appropriately for their clinical need, it is nonetheless a standard example of the range of data collected from most case note audits.

The clinical content of the nurse practitioner records research instrument was divided into two parts – Assessment, and Management/ Advice – with eight and five subscales respectively. For example, the 'Context and circumstances in which injury/illness occurred' is entered as 'Not recorded', 'Recorded without detail', 'Recorded in detail' or 'Not appropriate'. As this is a consultation study, it was felt that it would be a much more sensitive tool than that used by Dolan and Dale (1997), not least because it was looking for different information.

Conclusion

This chapter has looked at a range of theoretical and practical issues related to the development of this pilot study. These have included issues of access, ethics, sampling, the reliability and validity of research instruments, and the use and justification for use of the research instruments themselves. The next chapter will look at their administration and discuss whether they are fit for their purpose in the main study that, it is hoped, will follow.

Chapter 4
The pilot study

This chapter, describing the process of undertaking the pilot study, will be written in the form of a first-person narrative, because it may offer a richer description of what happened during the period of the research described. Qualitative researchers, such as Walford (1991) and Aamodt (1991), recommend the use of this 'thick description' when reporting research experiences. It will incorporate the methodological issues addressed in Chapter 3 and describe the practical challenges associated with undertaking what Robson (1994) describes as 'real-world research'.

Pilot study – practical challenges

Before describing the pilot study, it is important to highlight several aspects concerning my own role in this study. I am in receipt of a NHS Executive (South Thames) Research Training Fellowship, which has provided both the funding and the opportunity to explore the issue of nurse practitioner–patient consultation in some detail. I also have a fascination with understanding the ENP role and wish to make the consultation process more visible as a means of making more explicit why ENPs are perceived to be so successful and popular with patients.

Access

The first contact with the pilot site in question, which will be called Hawthorn Hospital, was in the summer of 1997 when I rang the senior ENP, 'James', to ask whether he would agree in principle for me to undertake a study into nurse practitioner–patient consultations. I had known James for a number of years and regarded him with a

35

mixture of respect and admiration for his achievements in the field of ENP care. As a nurse whom I would describe as an expert clinician as well as an articulate and highly regarded manager, I felt that his support would be crucial in gaining access to the pilot site.

I arranged to visit James a couple of weeks later, and outlined what at that time were fairly nebulous ideas to seek an understanding of the nurse practitioner–patient consultation. Among the reasons for approaching this PC/MIU rather than others was the fact that it had at that time no fewer than six ENPs working 12-hour shifts 7 days a week. This meant that there often two ENPs on duty at any time, which would, I anticipated, make the study easier to undertake. James was willing and supportive of the idea, and we arranged for me to meet other members of the ENP team to discuss it with them and gain their support and approval for the study. It was also agreed that it would be important to gain the approval of the (then Acting) Director of Nursing and the A&E clinical nurse manager. While the latter gave James considerable autonomy in his sphere of practice, it was nonetheless regarded as a professional courtesy to at least seek permission to undertake the study in this department, if only to make the nurse manager aware of my intended presence.

The meeting with the nurse practitioner team went well, and they made a number of invaluable suggestions that were incorporated into the study, for example the use of a radio-microphone attached to the ENP and connected by aerial to an audiotape for recording the consultation. This meant that the study itself reflected more accurately the actual practice of nurse practitioners, as I had origi-nally intended, rather than artificially constraining them to a desk, mimicking a GP consultation.

Having James as a sponsor certainly helped me to gain the trust of the ENPs, and my presence there may not have been possible without him. I was also facilitated by my track record as being one of the few nurse researchers, along with Dr Mike Walsh (for example, Walsh 1989, 1997), who had written about and undertaken research into ENPs' practice. This provided me with legitimacy and acceptance based on my experience of working with ENPs, and I also assured all of them that ethical approval would be sought and a copy of any subsequent reports or dissertation fed back to them.

The ENPs themselves had a wealth of experience in their field. All had undertaken the English National Board for Nursing, Health

Visiting and Midwifery (ENB) No. 3 course, 'Developing Autonomous Practice'. This is a six-month course that involves week-long periods in college, interspersed with practice placements learning the skills and knowledge required to become nurse practitioners. All of them had also undertaken the six-month ENB No. 199 'Accident and Emergency' course, which provides a grounding in the theory and practice of A&E nursing. Individually, they had worked in diverse A&E and MIUs, and in sick children's units, as well as abroad. When the unit opened in 1995, they also undertook a range of in-house study days with radiologists, microbiologists, ophthalmologists and so on in order to enable them to fulfil their expanded roles both effectively and efficiently.

The meeting with the Director of Nursing also included myself, the Senior Nurse for Research and Education for the hospital and James. I was aided in advance of the meeting by the generous comments of a nursing colleague who was undertaking a quite separate study in the hospital concerned. The Director of Nursing needed reassurances about the rationale for the study and why I had chosen this site, rather than another hospital. She made further valuable recommendations and put the Turkish language interpreter at my disposal in order to ensure that the views of this ethnic group were captured in the study. The Senior Nurse for Research and Education also offered to provide support for my application to the Local Research Ethics Committee (LREC), of which she was a member. In return, I offered to undertake a lecture on the future of nurse practitioners, based on work I was doing at that time. I also offered to contribute a £100 honorarium to the A&E department's education fund in recognition of the relatively small on-costs (i.e. additional costs incurred by the employer in relation to the employee) of my research to the organization. Access and acceptance gained, I appeared set for an early start for the study in late summer or early autumn 1997.

Gaining ethical approval

As noted in Chapter 3, the LREC required 34 copies of the application form. The Senior Nurse for Education was very generous in her support, but her workload meant that a day or two would go by between telephone calls to address queries. In addition to gaining the support of the LREC, I needed, as an employee at King's College

School of Medicine and Dentistry, a letter of confirmation that they would accept vicarious liability for my actions. This took some days to achieve as it was difficult to track down the Chair of the King's College Research Ethics Committee and convince him that qualitative research was a legitimate research tradition. While a handwritten fax supporting my research was forthcoming, it was another fortnight before a typed letter of approval was received that could be attached to the LREC application form.

In addition, some weeks passed before the Director of Nursing's letter of support arrived. This is meant not to reflect poorly on the individuals concerned, but to show that complex organizational structures, workload and holidays (this being the summer holiday period) meant that unexpected delays occurred. The LREC application form was sent by courier to the Ethics Committee Secretariat on the day that it was due in. It arrived one hour late, and the administrator refused to admit it for that month's meeting, thus imposing a minimum of 1 month's delay on gaining approval.

The meeting of the LREC to discuss my research application took place in October 1997, the results being posted to me a few days later. The application was rejected, but a number of helpful suggestions were made in order to make it acceptable. While the reasons for rejection were disappointing, they were nevertheless, for the most part, understandable, including the need to make it clear on forms for the patients that the study was a pilot, and to provide contact names and telephone numbers for patients who might have questions about the study when they went home. It would also be fair to suggest, however, that the questions on the application form itself reflected the positivistic bias of most health services research, for example calling participants 'subjects', and it was difficult to answer many of the Committee's questions in a meaningful way. Although this does not absolve my failure to gain approval on the first attempt, it does underline the need for a careful consideration of the LREC application form and of potential questions that might be voiced by the Committee. Indeed, while it is not usual practice for the applicant to be involved in the meeting, the absence resulting from annual leave commitments of the Senior Nurse for Research and Education cannot have helped my case.

In the event, the Chair of the LREC wrote advising me that if the Committee's conditions of acceptance were acted upon, he would exercise his discretion to approve the application using Chair's

Action without it having to come to the full committee again. By now it was late October, and I had started the time-taxing and intellectually demanding MSc in Educational Research Methodology at Oxford University. With the best of intentions, it was extremely difficult to juggle all the educational and research commitments, so I decided to concentrate on the coursework, advise James and his colleagues of my situation and submit my application again in the New Year, taking on board the various recommendations and directions of the LREC. The time lag also meant that the resubmitted research proposal was more rigorous in its attention to methodological detail, based largely on the knowledge gained during the course of the MSc, which I found was benefiting me enormously in terms of challenging many of my preconceptions about research theory and practice.

This time, research approval was awarded. However, because of a combination of examinations and other MSc course commitments, it was not possible to start the fieldwork until the summer of 1998. More positively, however, I was now, as a result of my course, far more familiar with the research and methodological processes attached to undertaking fieldwork. I also had greater confidence in my research abilities, which meant that I could concentrate on ensuring that the process was as rigorous as possible.

The patient's trajectory through the department

I arranged dates with the ENPs during which all of them would at some point be on duty while I was undertaking my fieldwork. In the interim, between my first meeting with them in the late summer of 1997 and undertaking my fieldwork in summer 1998, two of the ENPs had moved on to other positions, so instead of six ENPs there were now four, two of whom were working part-time hours. They were, however, no less generous in their time and commitment to the study.

The layout of the unit should be briefly explained. While the PC/MIU is part of the A&E department, it is a subunit with its own entrance and dedicated staff. There are six trolleys in one bay, and a desk and chair in another. In addition, there is an ophthalmic examination room for patients presenting with eye problems. While the ENPs work 12-hour shifts on the unit, they are assisted by A&E nursing staff who are assigned from the main department, as well as by postregistration A&E course students and preregistration nursing students on allocation.

Patients attending the A&E department are seen first by a triage nurse who assesses their condition, provides simple first aid and analgesia as appropriate, and determines their clinical priority based on the symptoms they describe. The patients may present with literally anything; it is the nurse's ability to gather information and make clinical judgements based on that information that determines the patient's trajectory through the A&E department (Mackway-Jones 1997). For example, it is critically important for the triage nurse to be able to ascertain whether the chest pain presented by a patient is cardiac or musculoskeletal in origin. Generally, however, most conditions that present to the A&E department are not life threatening; indeed, only 1 in 200 patients present with an immediately life-threatening condition such as cardiac arrest or multiple trauma (Audit Commission 1996).

Once the clinical priority, usually known as the triage category, of the patients has been identified, they will be asked to wait in the waiting room, or will be escorted through to the 'majors' side of A&E if their condition warrants more immediate attention or they need to lie down on a trolley. As most patients present with relatively minor conditions, such as lacerations and chest infections, they tend to wait, sometimes for several hours, in the waiting room. In the case of the PC/MIU, patients, and where appropriate their relatives, will be called through, a detailed consultation, examination, set of investigations and treatment then following. These are undertaken by the ENP or by the SHO, a junior medical doctor working for six months in A&E. Once treatment has been given, the patient is usually discharged, occasionally with a prescription for antibiotics in the case of infection, and/or is referred for further follow-up treatment by physiotherapists, their GP and so on as appropriate. Once called into the PC/MIU, the episode may last between half an hour and two hours depending on the need for investigations, the busyness of the department and other factors.

Finding a study sample

In order to ensure that patients were not placed under any undue pressure to agree to take part in the study, they were invited to speak to me if they were agreeable; this was done by the triage nurse, who was aware of the study and familiar with the inclusion and exclusion criteria. Nine patients declined to take part in the study, but it is important to stress that no one's care was in any way affected by their refusal. Reasons, when given, tended to be the perceived time constraints that the study would involve. When it was explained that the study would only delay their stay by approximately 10 minutes, some suggested that domestic commitments constrained them from waiting any longer than absolutely necessary. In most instances, however, no reason was offered or sought.

Where agreement to take part was given, the triage nurse identified the patient concerned, and I then introduced myself as 'Brian Dolan, a nurse researcher from King's College Hospital'. It was important for me to stress that I was a nurse as this, I believe, helped patients to have confidence that I was a health professional. I hoped that identifying my hospital base, rather than the university where I was studying, would also reassure potential respondents that I continued to work in a health service setting. I spent some time explaining the purpose of the research and going through the patient information leaflet I had written about the study. I then offered to leave the patient for a couple of minutes to read the leaflet. On my return, I asked the patient if there were any further questions and invited him or her to sign a patient consent form.

While this makes it sound easy, it was in practice anything but. I initially intended to get 5 or 6 patients per nurse practitioner, totalling 20–24 patients. In the event, over the space of 47 hours of fieldwork, 13 patients who met the inclusion criteria consented to take part in the study – an average of 1 patient every 3.6 hours. In the case of two consecutive 10-hour shifts, I managed to recruit only 3 patients in total. One of these days coincided with the first match of England's World Cup campaign. Although the number of accidents, illnesses and injuries might not necessarily be expected to decline during major sporting and cultural events, it is part of A&E folklore that a particularly good episode of a favourite television soap opera will see a temporary reduction in the number of patients attending A&E! These are not the things that one tends to read about in research methodology books.

For those patients who did agree to take part in the study, the process was as follows. Their consultation was audiotaped by the ENP, who had a radio-microphone attached to the lapel of his or her polo shirt, which, along with dark trousers, was the uniform. In order to reduce the Hawthorne effect, as well as for practical reasons, such as when the audiotape of one ENP was accidentally turned off, the first interviews were discarded, the data being collected from the second consultation onwards. Following the completion of the consultation with the ENP and immediately before discharge, the patient was invited to complete an MISS questionnaire, which took between 6 and 10 minutes depending on the patient. The patient was thanked for his or her involvement in the study, and left. The ENP then completed a post-consultation questionnaire. Once the case notes had been completed, their clinical content was then recorded on the clinical content of the nurse practitioner records audit sheet.

Field relations

'Fieldwork' refers to an investigation in which an observer maintains a face-to-face involvement with the members of a particular social setting for the purposes of scientific inquiry (Johnson 1976). In this instance, I was doing fieldwork in an environment with which I was very familiar, with ENPs whom I regarded with respect as peers and colleagues. While there was an initial feeling that having their consultation audiotaped seemed strange, all remarked how quickly they forgot the radio-microphone attached to them. They also expressed some surprise that the presence of the audiotaping did not appear to affect their consultation with patients, other than in terms of a passing reference to its presence to assure the patient that it was for the research about which they had already been told. The only other time that the research was referred to was at the end of the consultation, when the ENP asked the patient to come and see me about the MISS questionnaire.

In the early days of the fieldwork, a large number of questions were asked about my research, not just by the ENPs, but also by A&E doctors, staff nurses and postregistered students undertaking the A&E course. I had based myself at the nurses' station by the main six-bedded bay, where all the telephone, case note writing and other clerical activities occurred. My questionnaires, consent forms, audit forms and information sheets were available for anyone who wished to read them, and a number of staff chose to do so. This was intentional as I wished to be as open as was reasonably possible about my research activities. While Wolcott (1995) discusses the darker arts of fieldwork and the use of subterfuge to gain information, I saw little need to use such an approach. As professional colleagues, the ENPs were both trusting and trustworthy. As we all had respect for each other's roles, there was no sense of a hidden agenda on anyone's part.

I was also invited to join staff for coffee and lunch, being made to feel very welcome. There was no sense of being someone coming to 'check up on' the ENPs, and they expressed considerable interest in my application at that time to secure 2 more years' funding in order to undertake the main study. I was asked for advice on a range of professional issues and was, on a number of occasions, even asked for comments on patients' clinical conditions. That said, I never felt a sense of 'going native', a concern expressed in much of the ethnographic literature (Street 1992, Hammersley & Atkinson 1995, Ersser 1997): I was always a guest of the department rather than a part of it. This social and intellectual distance is necessary as a researcher, because, apart from the potential biases that can be introduced into the study without it, there is a need for critical analytic space to view the progress of the research more or less dispassionately.

The robustness of the research instruments

One of the main purposes of this pilot study was to test the instruments to be used. Whereas it is not appropriate to analyse the data from a pilot study in the conventional sense, it is appropriate to assess whether the instruments used are valid and reliable. This does not mean that what follows are findings, but means they should be interpreted as giving an indication of whether the chosen instruments would be suitable for use in the larger study that will follow.

The Multi-dimensional Interaction Scale

Charon et al (1994, p 955) have argued that:

> if one is to understand the enterprise of modern medicine, one must study medical discourse, examining the process and content of conversations between doctors and patients, the conversationalists goals, the context in which they speak, and ultimately the meanings that emerge from their interactions.

Using the MDIA instrument, a coder (in this case myself) analyses an interview directly from a transcription, listing topics sequentially and rating patient and nurse responsiveness within these topics on a coding sheet. As I listened to the audiotape, I recorded each topic as it was raised and noted whether it was raised by the ENP or patient. The microphone, although worn by the ENP, was sensitive enough to pick up the patient's voice too.

For purposes of analysis, each topic is assigned to a content category from a preselected list of categories. The MDIA currently lists 36 categories subdivided into five major content areas. The 'Biomedical' major content area lists such categories as prognosis, diagnostic procedures, medications and findings. 'Personal Habits' includes diet, exercise, alcohol and sex. The 'Psychosocial' major content area includes the health-care system, work and leisure activities, money, benefits, and family and significant others. The 'Patient–Nurse Relationship' area includes categories that focus on the nursing relationship. Although in the original publication, the latter content area focuses on the 'Patient–Doctor Relationship', this pilot study modified this to incorporate nursing rather than medical terminology. The fifth major content area is 'Other', which incorporates small talk and other information not relating to the consultation. As noted in the last chapter, both participants in the consultation can also be evaluated for their demonstration of such global characteristics as assertiveness or respectfulness. Finally, the consultation itself can be globally characterized using such descriptors as 'warm', 'trusting' and 'superficial'.

Horton and Bayne (1994) suggest listening to the audiotape, if possible, within 48 hours of recording. This was made somewhat easier as I was able to listen to the tapes in the car on the way home each evening. In the event, transcripts were also made of three of the six tapes, these being read and listened to several times. Although not strictly necessary, this was to reassure me that I could code from the audiotape and transcript with consistency.

At this point, it would probably be enlightening to provide one or two examples of the coding. One patient presented with an ankle injury. The ENP introduced himself, explained his role to the patient, outlined the patient's history as he understood it from the triage nurse, and asked the patient to tell him 'a little bit more about actually how you came to injure yourself'. There followed a series of questions concerning how the injury had occurred and how the patient managed it himself. Throughout the consultation, the ENP (coded ENP 01) scored highly on a 5-point Likert scale that included global scores such as 'Egalitarian–Condescending', Engaged–Abrupt', 'Respectful–Disrespectful' and 'Friendly–Hostile'.

The patient was asked whether he had put any ice on his ankle. When he replied that he had put it in warm water, the ENP did not accuse the patient of being wrong, instead suggesting 'Unfortunately, that's not the right thing to do' and then spending some time explaining the benefits of cold water for musculoskeletal injuries. The ENP scored well on the 'Biomedical' major content area of preventive measures. The MDIA also scores on compliments, shared laughter, the use of technical language and interruptions to the consultation. It appears to be a particularly helpful research instrument that captures quite well the interaction between nurse practitioner and patient.

The Medical Interview Satisfaction Scale

The MISS (Appendix III) measures satisfaction with a particular consultation as distinct from general attitudes towards nurses or health-care services. Wolfe et al (1978) believe that because the items in the MISS refer directly to a specific patient–provider interaction, this scale is likely to be more sensitive to actual differences in care than are measures of general attitudes.

The questionnaire was administered to the patients following their consultation with the ENP. This took approximately 6–10 minutes depending on the patient. I supplemented the written instructions on the front of the questionnaire with verbal instructions so that the patients would understand how to complete the questionnaire. They were then left alone to do this, being advised that if they had any further queries, I would be close by to assist. It was stressed that, for those patients who had relatives in attendance, only the patients should complete the questionnaire, and that they should not ask for help from their relatives. As they were generally within ear- and eyeshot of myself, it is fair to suggest that only the patients themselves completed the MISS, and the instructions, as well as the questionnaire itself, appeared to be well understood by them. Once they had completed the questionnaire, they were thanked for their contribution to the study and were free to leave the department.

The MISS itself has 26 items divided into three subscales: cognitive, affective and behavioural. Patients are asked to respond to statements such as 'The nurse practitioner told me the name of my problem in words I could understand' (cognitive), 'I felt this nurse practitioner accepted me as a person' (affective) and 'The nurse practitioner was too rough when she examined me' (behavioural). As the responses are measured on a 5-point Likert scale, the means and standard deviations of the nurses' scores could be measured both globally and for each subscale.

It was only during the writing-up phase of the work, after the MISS had been administered, that it was discovered that an error had been made in the Likert scales. In the original paper, Wolfe et al (1978) had included 'Agree' as one of the scales. This was erroneously excluded in the questionnaire administered to patients, consequently unbalancing the scale and forcing patients to choose between more strongly worded scales such as 'Strongly agree' or 'Strongly disagree'. This will be corrected in subsequent administrations of the research instrument.

ENPs scored highly on the subscales, meaning either that it is insufficiently sensitive, or that it perhaps reflects the patients' true level of satisfaction. This is more difficult to judge in the light of the oversight concerning the scale's recording, as outlined above. There is also an ongoing debate about the value of satisfaction scales, which this study is unlikely to fully resolve (Carr-Hill 1992, Williams 1994). However, given the validity and reliability of this research instrument as reported in other studies (for example, Stiles et al 1978), it seems a sufficiently sensitive research instrument for the purposes of the main study in this work.

Post-consultation nurse practitioner questionnaire

The purpose of this post-consultation questionnaire was to assess whether the ENP and patient felt similarly about consultation, comparing both the ENP and MISS questionnaires. Like the other elements of the pilot study, 13 questionnaires were returned. The information provided was cross-tabulated with the patient's identity number so that I could check whether the ENP's response appeared to reflect the patient's experience of the consultation (Appendix IV).

As well as details about the patients, such as their main presenting symptoms and diagnosis, the ENPs were asked how easy the consultation felt for them as both a nurse practitioner and an individual. They were asked to score this on a 5-point Likert scale from 'Totally straightforward' to 'Not at all straightforward'. The ENPs were also asked on a 5-Likert scale how relaxed they felt and how relaxed the patient seemed to feel. The scale ranged from 'Totally relaxed' to 'Not at all relaxed'. Four further questions – 'Did you feel there were any problems of communication? If so, what where they?', 'Was there anyone else present during the consultation?' and 'Are there any further comments you would like to make about this consultation?' – were also asked in this questionnaire.

In most instances, the ENPs scored 1 or 2 on the ease of the consultation, more frequently scoring a 2 on their own state of relaxation. In all four cases, the ENPs commented on being conscious of the audiotape. One commented, 'The 2 relates to the presence of tape but as this was a long interaction [with the patient], I relaxed after a while'. Another stated, '[The score of 2] was due to the presence of the tape but as the consultation lengthened I relaxed, forgot about it'. The ENPs were also asked to comment on how relaxed they felt the patient was. Again, in most instances, they scored a 1, but in some instances scored a 2, on the Likert scale, usually because of perceived language difficulties. Perhaps surprisingly, this did not appear to be reflected in the patient's own MISS questionnaire feedback, which suggests the patients were confident with their consultation with the ENP. It may also suggest a lack of cross-instrument sensitivity.

I am not convinced, on the basis of the administration of this instrument, that it is robust enough for use in the main study, and it does not seem sufficiently sensitive to address whether the ENP felt that the consultation went well. Open-ended questions on the consultation were frequently not answered, which could be due to its lack of perceived relevance or, which is perhaps more probable, to time pressure on the ENPs to see other patients. In the main study, it is likely to be replaced by a longer semi-structured interview investigating the ENP's role, the consultation process and its content, which will hopefully draw out issues such as how the ENP makes decisions, gains rapport with patients, makes them feel comfortable, gains relevant clinical information from them and provides health-promoting advice and psychosocial care.

Audit of clinical content of nurse practitioner records

This was undertaken after the ENPs had completed their case notes.

The ENPs were good at recording the biomedical details of patients' presenting problems, and their management. However, it was clear that the case notes do not reflect the amount of health-promotion input given to the patient. This suggests that, as an index of quality, clinical case notes are a poor instrument. The discriminators of assessment and management/advice given, that is 'Recorded in detail' and 'Recorded without detail' led to rather arbitrary judgements being made about what 'detail' implied, so more work is needed to fine-tune these. Otherwise, this is a useful research instrument, if only to highlight the invisibility of much of nursing practice that goes on behind the screens (Lawlor 1991) (Appendix V).

Conclusion

This chapter has considered some of the practical issues and challenges associated with doing real-world research. It has described the research process, and discussed the various research instruments used and whether they appeared to be robust enough to be used in a larger-scale study. It would appear that the MDIA and MISS tools work well and do not need further refinement. The post-consultation questionnaire, however, is not sufficiently reliable and valid to be particularly useful, and the clinical content of case notes audit tool may need fine-tuning in terms of definitions of recording, although its administration appeared to be unproblematic.

The final chapter will draw together again the theoretical and practical dimensions of this study, highlight the lessons learned and reiterate the research questions before asking whether this pilot study has answered them successfully enough for a larger-scale study to be carried out.

Chapter 5
Conclusion

This has been an interesting and informative exercise that will be an invaluable help in the next phase of this research. It is not the purpose of a pilot study to be analysed, so the conclusion will concentrate on methodological issues rather than findings. Van Ort (1981) contends that a pilot study is conducted for one or more of the following reasons:

- to determine the feasibility of a major study;
- to identify problems in the research design;
- to refine the data collection and analysis plan;
- to test the instrument(s) to be used in a major study;
- to give the researcher some experience with the subjects, methodology and instruments.

Using Van Ort's (1981) criteria as a template, it is worth evaluating whether these have been met. Based on the information provided by the literature, process and application of the research instruments, it does appear that this study could be undertaken on a larger scale. Problems with the research have been identified, not least in the sampling, given the relatively lengthy periods required to recruit participants among the patient population. The data collection and analysis was somewhat hampered by the sampling matters outlined above, suggesting that other approaches should be considered. The data analysis, albeit complex because of its multiple sources, presented fewer challenges than anticipated, which was quite reassuring.

The instruments in the study, subject to fine-tuning where appropriate, appear to be sufficiently robust to be used in a larger-scale study. The Post-consultation nurse practitioner questionnaire has problems and will be discarded in favour of a semi-structured interview, which will be developed and piloted before being introduced in the larger study. Finally, the piloting experience itself has been invaluable in providing valuable insights into participant recruitment, methodological challenges and instrument administration issues that might not otherwise have been considered.

It is worth reiterating the aims, objectives and research questions in order to assess whether it has achieved its intentions. This pilot study aimed:

- To analyse the process and content of nurse practitioner consultations and appraise patient satisfaction in A&E departments.

Its objectives were:

- To test a research tool to describe the nurse practitioner consultation process and content in an A&E department.
- To test a research tool to describe the nurse practitioner's perceptions of the consultation.
- To test a research tool to assess patient satisfaction with nurse practitioner consultations.
- To test a research tool to audit the case notes of nurse practitioner consultations.

The research questions were:

- What are the process and content of ENP consultations in A&E departments and MIUs?
- How do ENP and patient perceptions about the consultation process compare in A&E departments and MIUs in terms of satisfaction?
- How does the nurse practitioner's documentation of the consultation compare with a structured analysis of the consultation's process and content?

With the exception of the post-consultation nurse practitioner questionnaire, the research instruments tested seem sufficiently robust to be used in the main study. This does not mean they were not without limitations or could not benefit from further fine-tuning, as was seen particularly with the clinical content of the nurse practitioner records audit tool. The strengths and difficulties associated with the various research instruments have been considered in detail in Chapter 4. An additional approach, that of a semi-structured interview, will seek to explore some of the range of issues confronting ENPs in their consultations.

The literature review in Chapter 2 suggested a paucity of studies looking exclusively at nurse practitioner–patient consultations. Instead, the focus of most studies of nurse practitioners in the UK have tended to be comparative (usually with junior medical staff) or evaluative within the wider health-care system. Although these are undoubtedly valuable in assessing the effectiveness and efficiency of the service and care delivery, they fail to address the added value that nurse practitioners bring to the patient's experience. The proposed study will attempt to redress that balance, at least a little.

Ford and Walsh (1994) argue that the development of the nurse practitioner offers great potential for nursing, but it may also fall into the trap of becoming ritualistic practice if nursing does not control the educational process for nurse practitioners, and if their role becomes circumscribed by a mass of arbitrary rules and regulations. In addition, the external forces impacting on ENPs, for example health services reforms, changing roles and relationships with medical personnel, reductions in junior doctors' hours, improving educational opportunities and so on, may leave little space for them to reflect on and consolidate their practice.

Patterson and Haddad (1992, p 20) propose that:

> nurse practitioners are those nurses who push beyond the boundaries of their profession; who have the vision and flexibility necessary to consider new possibilities for improvement and/or expansion; who have the urge to ask questions and seek out the answers; who are willing to take risks and face challenges associated with breaking new ground; and who have the ability to articulate their thoughts clearly as they move ahead such that they contribute to the understanding and development of new knowledge and skills within nursing and thus lead their profession forward to meet the needs and demands of society.

The evidence presented in this pilot study suggests this position still remains some way off as ENPs in the UK become more established and their role becomes more clearly defined and understood. It is the aim of the subsequent study to assist in helping to clarify that definition and understanding.

References

Aamodt AM (1991) Ethnography and epistemology: generating nursing knowledge. In Morse JM (Ed.) Qualitative Nursing Research: A Contemporary Dialogue. Newbury Park, CA: Sage.

Abbott P, Sapsford R (1998) Research Methods for Nurses and the Caring Professions. Buckingham: Open University Press.

Adelman RD, Greene MG, Charon R (1991) Issues in physician–elderly patient interaction. Ageing Society 11: 127–48.

Arborelius E, Bremberg S (1992) What can doctors do to achieve a successful consultation?: videotaped interviews analysed by the 'consultation map' method. Family Practice 9(1): 61–6.

Audit Commission (1996) By Accident or Design: Improving A&E Services in England and Wales. London: HMSO.

Baker R (1990) Development of a questionnaire to assess patients' satisfaction with consultations in general practice. British Journal of General Practice 40: 487–90.

Baker R (1996) Characteristics of practices, general practitioners and patients related to levels of patients' satisfaction with consultations. British Journal of General Practice 46: 601–5.

Beisecker AE, Beisecker TD (1990) Patient information-seeking behaviors when communicating with doctors. Medical Care 28(1): 19–28.

Benton D, Cormack DFS (1996) Gaining access to the research site. In Cormack DFS (Ed.) The Research Process in Nursing, 3rd Edn. Oxford: Blackwell Science, pp 102–10.

Bliss A (1976) Quoted in Nurse Practitioner (1985) A look back. Nurse Practitioner 10 (10): 15–19 (Editorial).

Bowling A (1997) Research Methods in Health: Investigating Health and Health Services. Buckingham: Open University Press.

Brykczynski KA (1993) Response to 'Nurse practitioner–patient discourse: uncovering the voice of nursing in primary care practice'. Scholarly Inquiry for Nursing Practice 7(3): 159–63.

Burgess R (1984) In the Field: An Introduction to Field Research. London: Routledge.

Burgess R (1990) Sponsors, gatekeepers, members and friends. In Shaffir W (Ed.) Experiencing Fieldwork: An Introduction to Field Research. Newbury Park; CA: Sage.

Butler NM, Campion PD, Cox AD (1992) Exploration of doctor and patient agendas in general practice consultations. Social Science and Medicine 35(9): 1145–55.

Byrne GS (1992) The accident and emergency department: nurses' priorities and patients' anxieties. Unpublished PhD thesis, University of Northumbria.

Byrne G, Heyman R (1997) Understanding nurses' communication with patients in accident and emergency departments using a symbolic interactionist perspective. Journal of Advanced Nursing 26: 93–100.

Byrne PS, Heath CC (1980) Practitioners' use of non-verbal behaviour in real consultations. Journal of the Royal College of General Practitioners 30: 327–31.

Carr-Hill R (1992) The measurement of patient satisfaction. Journal of Public Health Medicine 14(3): 236–49.

Casey N (1996) Editorial. Nursing Standard 10(43): 1.

Cassell EJ, Skopek L, Fraser B (1977) A preliminary model for the examination of doctor–patient communication. Language Science 43: 10–13.

Chambers N (1996) Nurse practitioners in primary care: an alternative to a consultation with the doctor? Unpublished PhD thesis, University of Manchester.

Chambers N (1998) Nurse Practitioners in Primary Care. Oxford: Radcliffe Medical Press.

Charon R, Greene MG, Adelman RD (1994) Multi-Dimensional Interaction Analysis: a collaborative approach to the study of medical discourse. Social Science and Medicine 39(7): 955–65.

Cohen L, Manion L (1994) Research Methods in Education, 4th Edn. London: Routledge.

Cole F, Ramirez E, Mickanin J (1998) ENP education: a United States perspective. Emergency Nurse 6(4): 12–14.

Cooper M, Robb A (1996) Nurse Practitioners in A&E: a literature review. Emergency Nurse 4(3): 19–22.

Dale J (1992) Primary Care in A and E: Establishing the Service. The Accident and Emergency Primary Care Project. London: King's College School of Medicine and Dentistry.

Dale J, Dolan B (1996) Do patients use minor injury units appropriately? Journal of Public Health 18(2): 152–6.

Dale J, Green J, Glucksman E, Higgs R(1991) Providing for Primary Care: Progress in A&E. London: Department of General Practice, King's College School of Medicine and Dentistry.

Dale J, Morley V, Dolan B (1996) An Evaluation of A&E/Primary Care Service Developments in West London for Ealing, Hounslow and Hammersmith Health Agency. London: King's College School of Medicine and Dentistry.

Diers D, Molde S (1979) Some conceptual and methodological issues in nurse practitioner research. Research in Nursing and Health 2: 73–84.

Dolan B (1993) Gender and change. In Project 2000: Reflection and Celebration. (Ed. B Dolan) London: Scutari Press.

Dolan B, Dale J (1997) Characteristics of self referred patients attending minor injury units. Journal of Accident and Emergency Medicine 14: 212–14.

Dolan B, Dale J, Morley V (1997) Nurse practitioners: the role in A&E and primary care. Nursing Standard 11(17): 33–8.

Donabedian A (1968) Promoting quality through evaluating the process of care. Medical Care 6: 181–202.

Dunn L (1997) A literature review of advanced clinical practice in the United States of America. Journal of Advanced Nursing 25: 814–19.

Eisner EW (1991) The Enlightened Eye: Qualitative Inquiry and the Enhancement of Educational Practice. New York: Macmillan.

Ersser S (1997) Nursing as a Therapeutic Activity: An Ethnography. Aldershot: Avebury.

Fawcett-Henesy A (1991) The British Scene. In J Salvage (Ed). Nurse Practitioners: Working for Change in Primary Health Care Nursing. London: King's Fund Centre, pp 44–50.

Foddy W (1994) Constructing Questions for Interviews and Questionnaires: Theory and Practice in Social Research. Cambridge: Cambridge University Press.

Ford P, Walsh M (1994) New Rituals for Old: Nursing through the Looking Glass. Oxford: Butterworth-Heinemann.

Ford-Gilboe M, Campbell J, Berman H (1995) Stories and numbers: coexistence without compromise. Advances in Nursing Sciences 18(1): 14–26.

Foster P (1996) Observational research. In Sapsford R, Jupp V (Eds) Data Collection and Analysis. London: Sage, pp 57–93.

Freeman B, Negrete VF, Davis M, Korsch BM (1971) Gaps in doctor–patient communication: doctor–patient interaction analysis. Pediatric Research 5: 298–311.

Freij RM, Duffy T, Hackett D, Cunningham D, Fothergill J (1996) Radiographic interpretation by nurse practitioners in a minor injuries unit. Journal of Accident and Emergency Medicine 13(1): 41–3.

Geolet D (1975) The emergency nurse practitioner. Nurse Practitioner 1(12): 28.

Goodwin LD, Goodwin WL (1984) Qualitative vs. quantitative research or qualitative and quantitative research? Nursing Research 33: 378–80.

Greene MG, Hoffman S, Charon R, Adelman R (1987) Psychosocial concerns in the medical encounter: a comparison of the interactions of doctors with their old and young patients. Gerontologist 27: 164–8.

Guba E (1981) Criteria for assessing the trustworthiness of naturalistic inquiries. Educational Communication and Technology Journal 29(2): 75–91.

Hammersley M, Atkinson P (1995) Ethnography: Principles in Practice, 2nd Edn. London: Routledge.

Hayden ML, Richter Davies L, Clore ER (1982) Facilitators and inhibitors of the emergency nurse practitioner role. Nursing Research 31(5): 294–9.

Head S (1988) Nurse practitioners: the new pioneers. Nursing Times 84(26): 27–8.

Heartfield M (1996) Nursing documentation and nursing practice: a discourse analysis. Journal of Advanced Nursing 24: 98–103.

Henbest RJ, Stewart M (1990) Patient-centredness in the consultation. 2: Does it really make a difference? Family Practice 7: 28–33.

Hicks C, Hennessy C (1998) A triangulation approach to the identification of acute sector nurses' training needs for formal nurse practitioner status. Journal of Advanced Nursing 27: 117–31.

Horton I, Bayne R (1994) Some guidelines on the use of audio-tape recordings in counsellor education and training. Counselling (Aug): 213–14.

Howie P (1992) Development of the nurse practitioner. Nursing Standard 6: 10–11.

James MR, Pyrgos N (1989) Nurse practitioners in the accident and emergency department. Archives of Accident and Emergency Medicine 6: 241–6.

Jarrett N, Payne S (1995) A selective review of the literature on nurse–patient communication: has the patient's contribution been neglected? Journal of Advanced Nursing 22(1): 72–8.

Johnson JM (1976) Doing Field Research. New York: Free Press.

Johnson R (1993) Nurse practitioner–patient discourse: uncovering the voice of nursing in primary care practice. Scholarly Inquiry for Nursing Practice 7(3): 143–57.

Korsch BM, Gozzi EK, Francis V (1968) Gaps in doctor–patient communication. 1: Doctor–patient interaction and patient satisfaction. Pediatrics 42(5): 855–69.

Lawlor J (1991) Behind the Screens: Nursing, Somology, and the Problem of the Body. Edinburgh: Churchill Livingstone.

LeCompte MD, Goetz JP (1982) Problems of reliability and validity in ethnographic research. Review of Educational Research 52(1): 31–60.

Lynaugh J, Bates B (1973) The two languages of nursing and medicine. American Journal of Nursing 73(1): 66–9.

McKenna H (1994) The Delphi technique: a worthwhile research approach for nursing? Journal of Advanced Nursing 19: 1221–5.

Mackway-Jones K (1997) Emergency Triage. London: BMJ Publishing Group.

Marshall J, Edwards C, Lambert M (1997) Administration of medicines by emergency nurse practitioners according to protocols in an accident and emergency department. Journal of Accident and Emergency Medicine 14: 233–7.

Mauksch L (1987) The nurse practitioner movement. American Journal of Public Health 68: 1074–5.

Meek SJ, Ruffles G, Anderson G, Ohiorenoya D (1995) Nurse practitioners in accident and emergency departments: a national survey. Journal of Accident and Emergency Medicine 12: 177–81.

Meek SJ, Ruffles G, Anderson G, Ohiorenoya D (1998) Can A&E nurse practitioners interpret radiographs?: a multicentre study. Journal of Accident and Emergency Medicine 15: 105–7.

Mitchell C (1983) Case and situation analysis. Sociological Analysis 31(2): 187–211.

Morris F, Head S, Holkar V (1989) The nurse practitioner: help in clarifying clinical and educational activities in Accident and Emergency Departments. Health Trends 21: 124–6.

Moser CA, Kalton G (1971) Survey Methods in Social Investigation, 2nd Edn. Aldershot: Dartmouth.

National Institute for Nursing (1993) Code of Conduct for Researchers. Oxford: National Institute for Nursing.

Oakley A (1984) The importance of being a nurse. Nursing Times (12 Dec): 24–7.

Patterson C, Haddad B (1992) The advanced nurse practitioner: common attributes. Canadian Journal of Nursing Administration (Nov/Dec): 19–22.

Pendleton D (1983) Doctor–patient communication: a review. In Pendleton D, Hasler J (Eds) Doctor–patient Communication. London: Academic Press, pp 5–55.

Poulton B (1996) Use of the consultation satisfaction questionnaire to examine patients' satisfaction with general practitioners and community nurses: reliability, replicability and discriminant validity. British Journal of General Practice 46: 26–31.

Prescott PA, Driscoll L (1979) Issues in evaluation of nurse practitioner effectiveness: a comparison of physician–nurse practitioner comparison studies. Evaluating Health Professions 2(4): 387–418.

Prescott PA, Driscoll L (1980) Evaluating nurse practitioner performance. Nurse Practitioner (Jul/Aug): 28–32.

Prescott PA, Jacox A, Collar M, Goodwin L (1981) The nurse practitioner rating form. Part I: Conceptual development and potential uses. Nursing Research 30(4): 223–8.

Read SM, George S (1994) Nurse practitioner in accident and emergency departments: reflections on a pilot study. Journal of Advanced Nursing 19: 705–16.

Reveley S (1998) The role of the triage nurse practitioner in general practice: an analysis of the role. Journal of Advanced Nursing 28(3): 584–91.

Risser HL (1975) Development of an instrument to measure patient satisfaction with nurses and nursing care in primary settings. Nursing Research 24: 45–52.

Robson C (1994) Real World Research: A Resource for Social Scientists and Practitioner-researchers. Oxford: Blackwell.

Roter DL (1989) Studies of doctor–patient interaction. Annual Review of Public Health 10: 163–80.

Roter D, Frankel R (1992) Quantitative and qualitative approaches to the evaluation of medical dialogue. Social Science and Medicine 34(10): 1097–103.

Royal College of Nursing (1992) Emergency Nurse Practitioners: Guidance from the Royal College of Nursing Accident and Emergency Nursing Association and Emergency Nurse Practitioners' Special Interest Group. London: RCN.

Royal College of Nursing (1996) Emergency Nurse Practitioners: Position Statement. London: RCN.

Royal College of Nursing (1998) Research Ethics: Guidance for Nurses Involved in Research or any Investigative Project Involving Human Subjects. London: RCN.

Salisbury CJ, Tettersell MJ. (1988) Comparison of the work of a nurse practitioner with that of a general practitioner. Journal of the Royal College of General Practitioners 38: 314–16.

Schofield JW (1993) Increasing the generalisability of qualitative research. In Hammersley M (Ed.) Educational Research: Current Issues. London: Paul Chapman, pp 91–114.

Schultz PR (1992) Attending to many voices: beyond the qualitative–quantitative dialectic. Communicating Nursing Research 25: 73–83.

Shih FJ (1998) Triangulation in nursing research: issues of conceptual clarity and purpose. Journal of Advanced Nursing 28(3): 631–41.

Skopek L (1979) Doctor–patient conversation: a way of analysing its linguistic problems. Semiotica 98: 301–11.

South East Thames Regional Health Authority (1994) Standards for A&E Practice (Revised Edition). Bexhill-on-Sea: SETRHA.

Stanford D (1987) Nurse practitioner research: issues in practice and theory. Nurse Practitioner 12(1): 64–75.

Stiles WB, Putnam SM, Wolf MH, James SA (1978) Interaction exchange structure and patient satisfaction with medical interviews. Medical Care 17: 667–81.

Stilwell B (1985) Oportunities in general practice. Nursing Mirror 161(19): 30–1.

Stilwell B (1991) An ideal consultation. In Salvage J (Ed.) Nurse Practitioners: Working for Change in Primary Health Care Nursing. London: King's Fund Centre.

Stilwell B, Greenfield, Drury M, Hull FM (1987) A nurse practitioner in general practice: working style and pattern of consultations. Journal of the Royal College of General Practitioners 37: 154–7.

Street AF (1992) Inside Nursing: A Critical Ethnography of Clinical Nursing Practice. New York: State University of New York Press.

Tye CC (1997) The emergency nurse practitioner role in major accident and emergency departments: professional issues and the research agenda. Journal of Advanced Nursing 26: 364–70.

UKCC (United Kingdom Central Council for Nursing, Midwifery and Health Visiting) (1998) A Higher Level of Practice: Consultation Document. London: UKCC.

Van Ort S (1981) Research designs: pilot study. In Krampitz SD, Pavlovich N (Eds) Readings for Nursing Research. St Louis, MO: CV Mosby, pp 49–53.

Vuori H, Aaku T, Aine E, Erkko R, Johansson RC (1972) Doctor–patient relationships in the light of patients' experiences. Social Science and Medicine 6: 723–36.

Walford G (1991) Doing Educational Research. London: Routledge.

Walsh M (1989) The A&E department and the nurse practitioner. Nursing Standard 4(11): 34–5.

Walsh M (1997) Commentary: nurse practitioner role should be explicitly defined. Nursing Standard 11(17): 33–8.

Williams B (1994) Patient satisfaction: a valid concept? Social Science and Medicine 38(4): 509–16.

Wolcott HF (1995) The Art of Fieldwork. Walnut Creek, CA: AltaMira Press.

Wolfe MH, Putnam SM, James SA, Stiles WB (1978) The medical interview satisfaction scale: development of a scale to measure patient perceptions of physician behaviour. Journal of Behavioural Medicine 1: 391–401.

Wood KM (1979) Nurse–patient communication in an accident department. Unpublished MSc dissertation, Manchester University.

Yin RK (1994) Case Study Research: Design and Methods, 2nd Edn. Thousand Oaks, CA: Sage.

Appendix I
Patient Consent Form

Dear Patient

HOSPITAL PRIMARY CARE/MINOR INJURIES UNIT
CONSENT FORM

I am conducting a survey of the nurse practitioner service that is currently offered here, in order to discover whether there are any further improvements that could be made. I would appreciate your help.

If you are willing to help, I would be very grateful if you would allow your consultation with the nurse practitioner to be recorded on a tape-recorder. The recording will not interfere with your treatment, and apart from the nurse practitioner and yourself or your relative(s), no one else will be present when the audiotaping takes place.

When you have finished seeing the nurse practitioner, would you please answer a short questionnaire. The questionnaire will take approximately 4–5 minutes to complete.

Please return the questionnaire in the attached envelope to me when you have completed it. Neither the nurse practitioners nor the doctors will know what answers you have given, and your response will remain strictly confidential. The tapes will be kept safely under lock and key, and once the study has been completed the tapes will be destroyed.

If you do not wish to participate at all, please return your uncompleted questionnaire to the receptionist or nursing staff. This will not affect your treatment in any way.

If you have any questions please do not hesitate to speak to —, Nurse Researcher on —, or —, Senior Nurse Practitioner on —.

Thank you very much for your time and help.

Yours sincerely

Nurse Researcher

HOSPITAL PRIMARY CARE/MINOR INJURIES UNIT
CONSENT FORM

I have given my consent to having my consultation with the nurse practitioner recorded on audiotape. I understand that once the study has been completed the audiotapes will be destroyed.

I also agree to complete a questionnaire following my consultation with the nurse practitioner. The reasons for the study have been explained to me and I understand them.

I understand that the information provided by me will be treated in the strictest confidence, that I can withdraw my consent to taking any further part in the study at any time and this will not affect my treatment in any way.

Signature

Name in block capitals

Appendix II
Patient Information Leaflet

An analysis of nurse practitioner consultations and patient satisfaction in A & E departments and minor injuries units.

Information for participants in a research project

We invite you to take part in a pilot research study that we think may be important. The information that follows tells you about it. It is important that you understand what is in the leaflet. It says what will happen if you take part and what the risks might be. Try to make sure that you know what will happen to you if you decide to take part. Whether or not you do take part is entirely your choice. Please ask any questions you want to about the research, and we will try our best to answer them. **You do not have to take part in this study, and if you do not wish to do so, it will not affect your treatment in any way.**

Q. Why have you been asked to take part in this research?

We are approaching patients who are attending the Minor Injuries Unit for treatment by a nurse practitioner. This is the pilot phase of a larger study that will begin later this year.

Q. What is the goal of the research?

We wish to find out how a nurse practitioner manages patient consultations and to examine patient satisfaction with the nurse practitioners. In the pilot phase, the questionnaires for examining these points are being tested for use in a larger study.

Q. What does involvement in the study mean for you?

Your consultation with the nurse practitioner will be audiotaped, and you are free to ask for recording to be stopped at any time. You will also be invited to complete a questionnaire at the end of your consultation. All information will only be used by the researcher and will not be seen by the nurse practitioners.

Q. Will taking part in this medical research be of specific benefit to you?

While there will be no 'medical' benefit to you, it is hoped that this study will help nurse practitioners to understand how they deal with patients and find out how satisfied patients are with the service.

Q. Will you have to come back to the Primary Care/Minor Injuries Unit as part of the research?

No.

Q. Are there any potential hazards for you taking part in the research?

None at all. You will receive the same treatment and advice as you would ordinarily have done.

Q. Are there any factors that would exclude you from taking part in this research?

There are age limitations and urgency of condition, which would exclude us from approaching particular patients, but we do not feel that you fall into any of our exclusion categories.

Q. How will the confidentiality of your medical condition be protected?

The only people to have access to the tape-recording of your conversation with the nurse practitioner will be the researcher and the administrator, who are bound by the terms of the Data Protection Act. Recordings will be locked away in secure conditions. The recordings will be given a code number so that your name will not be known.

Q. Whom should you contact if you are concerned or need more information about the study?

The lead researcher is —, who is Nursing Research Fellow at the Department of General Practice and Primary Care, King's College School of Medicine and Dentistry.
He can be contacted on —.
— Senior Nurse Practitioner, Primary Care/Minor Injuries Unit, is also available on —. Both will be very happy to answer any queries you may have.

Appendix III
Medical Interview Satisfaction Scale

Primary care/minor injuries unit pilot study of nurse practitioner consultations

AFTER YOU HAVE SEEN THE NURSE PRACTITIONER:

On the left hand side of the page you will see certain statements which refer to the *consultation you have just had with the nurse practitioner.*

Please circle around the words on the right that indicate how you feel about the statements on the left.

For example:

The nurse practitioner was kind to me today	Strongly Disagree	Disagree	Uncertain	Strongly Agree	Not Applicable

If you feel that the nurse practitioner was kind, you might put a circle around the words 'Strongly Agree'. If you feel that the nurse practitioner was not kind, you might out a circle around the words 'Disagree' *or* 'Strongly Disagree'. If you feel that the statement is not applicable to your consultation, please put a circle around the words 'Not Applicable'.

Please answer the following questions about the consultation you have just had. Please answer <u>all</u> of the questions and be sure to answer them carefully as we have had to reverse the order of some of the words.

Thank you very much for your help.

Example

The nurse practitioner was kind to me today	Strongly Disagree	Disagree	(Uncertain)	Strongly Agree	Not Applicable

NOW PLEASE ANSWER THE QUESTIONS.

After talking to the nurse practitioner, I have a good idea about the changes to expect in my health over the next few days and weeks	Strongly Disagree	Disagree	Uncertain	Strongly Agree	Not Applicable
After talking to the nurse practitioner, I felt much better about my problems	Strongly Disagree	Disagree	Uncertain	Strongly Agree	Not Applicable
I was satisfied with the nurse practitioner's decision about the medicines I should or should not take	Strongly Disagree	Disagree	Uncertain	Strongly Agree	Not Applicable
The nurse practitioner examined me thoroughly	Strongly Disagree	Disagree	Uncertain	Strongly Agree	Not Applicable
The nurse practitioner was too rough when he/she examined me	Strongly Disagree	Disagree	Uncertain	Strongly Agree	Not Applicable
The nurse practitioner told me the name of my problem in words I could understand	Strongly Disagree	Disagree	Uncertain	Strongly Agree	Not Applicable
I felt that this nurse practitioner accepted me as a person	Strongly Disagree	Disagree	Uncertain	Strongly Agree	Not Applicable
The nurse practitioner told me how my problem would affect my ability to work	Strongly Disagree	Disagree	Uncertain	Strongly Agree	Not Applicable
I feel that I understand pretty well the nurse practitioner's plan for helping	Strongly Disagree	Disagree	Uncertain	Strongly Agree	Not Applicable
The nurse practitioner I saw today would be someone I would trust with my life	Strongly Disagree	Disagree	Uncertain	Strongly Agree	Not Applicable
The nurse practitioner gave me a chance to say what was really on my mind	Strongly Disagree	Disagree	Uncertain	Strongly Agree	Not Applicable

After talking to the nurse practitioner, I now know how serious my problem is	Strongly Disagree	Disagree	Uncertain	Strongly Agree	Not Applicable
The nurse practitioner gave instructions too fast during my consultation	Strongly Disagree	Disagree	Uncertain	Strongly Agree	Not Applicable
The nurse practitioner really understood how I felt about my problem	Strongly Disagree	Disagree	Uncertain	Strongly Agree	Not Applicable
I really felt understood by my nurse practitioner	Strongly Disagree	Disagree	Uncertain	Strongly Agree	Not Applicable
The nurse practitioner seemed to know what he/she was doing	Strongly Disagree	Disagree	Uncertain	Strongly Agree	Not Applicable
I felt free to talk to the nurse practitioner about my private thoughts	Strongly Disagree	Disagree	Uncertain	Strongly Agree	Not Applicable
The nurse practitioner was not friendly to me	Strongly Disagree	Disagree	Uncertain	Strongly Agree	Not Applicable
The nurse practitioner looked into all the problems I mentioned	Strongly Disagree	Disagree	Uncertain	Strongly Agree	Not Applicable
The nurse practitioner has relieved my worries about being seriously ill	Strongly Disagree	Disagree	Uncertain	Strongly Agree	Not Applicable
I feel that the nurse practitioner did not spend enough time with me	Strongly Disagree	Disagree	Uncertain	Strongly Agree	Not Applicable
The nurse practitioner told me what the medicines he/she had prescribed would do for me	Strongly Disagree	Disagree	Uncertain	Strongly Agree	Not Applicable
I felt that the nurse practitioner did not take my problems very seriously	Strongly Disagree	Disagree	Uncertain	Strongly Agree	Not Applicable

I felt that the nurse practitioner was very good at explaining the reasons for tests, such as X-rays	Strongly Disagree	Disagree	Uncertain	Strongly Agree	Not Applicable

I felt relaxed during this consultation	Strongly Disagree	Disagree	Uncertain	Strongly Agree	Not Applicable

Did the nurse practitioner give you a prescription?	(please circle your response)	Yes	No

Did you want a prescription?	(please circle your response)	Yes	No

Did the nurse practitioner give you a full examination of your illness/injury?	(please circle your response)	Yes	No

Did you want a full examination of your illness/injury?	(please circle your response)	Yes	No

Did you feel tense during the consultation?	Yes	No

Overall, how satisfied were you with your consultation?	Extremely Satisfied	Moderately Satisfied	Uncertain	Moderately Dissatisfied	Extremely Dissatisfied

If you have any comments you would like to make about these questions, please write them here.

Thank you very much for your help

Appendix IV
Post-consultation Nurse Practitioner Questionnaire

POST-CONSULTATION NURSE PRACTITIONER QUESTIONNAIRE

Patient ID number ....

Please complete one of these questionnaires *after* you have seen the patient.

Nurse Practitioner ID number ....

Patient:
1.   Male/Female
2.   Age/Date of birth
3.   Main symptoms presented

4.   Diagnosis

5.   Have you treated this patient before? (please circle response)   YES/NO
6.   How easy was this consultation for <u>you</u> to deal with?
     a. As a nurse practitioner (please circle number)

     Totally   1   2   3   4   5   Not at all
     straightforward   straightforward

     b. As an individual (please circle number)

     Totally   1   2   3   4   5   Not at all
     straightforward   straightforward

7.   How relaxed did you feel? (please circle a number)

     Totally relaxed   1   2   3   4   5   Not at all
                                                     relaxed

8.   How relaxed was the patient? (please circle a number)

     Totally relaxed   1   2   3   4   5   Not at all
                                                     relaxed

9.   Did you feel that there were any problems of communication? If so what
       were they?

10.   Was anyone else present during this consultation?

11.   Are there any further comments that you would like to make about this
       consultation?

Thank you for completing this questionnaire

Appendix V
Clinical Content of Nurse Practitioner Records

CLINICAL CONTENT OF NURSE PRACTITIONER RECORDS

A&E number ☐ ☐ ☐ ☐ ☐ ☐　　　Date: ☐ ☐ ☐ ☐ ☐ ☐

Nurse practitioner code　　☐ ☐　　　　A&E record:
Nurse practitioner's name
0 = not recorded　　1 = recorded　☐

ASSESSMENT: PRESENTING PROBLEM(S):

1. Context and circumstances in which injury/illness occurred
   0 = Not recorded　　1 = Recorded without detail　2 = Recorded in detail
   X = Not appropriate　　　　　　　　　　　　　　　　　　　　　☐

2. Expectations and beliefs about care/treatment required
   0 = Not recorded　　1 = Recorded without detail　2 = Recorded in detail
   X = Not appropriate　　　　　　　　　　　　　　　　　　　　　☐

3. Relevant past medical history/co-existing problems
   0 = Not recorded　　1 = Recorded without detail　2 = Recorded in detail
   X = Not appropriate　　　　　　　　　　　　　　　　　　　　　☐

4. Lifestyle/risk factors (smoking, alcohol, drugs, etc)
   0 = Not recorded　　1 = Recorded without detail　2 = Recorded in detail
   X = Not appropriate　　　　　　　　　　　　　　　　　　　　　☐

5. Home/family circumstances
   0 = Not recorded　　1 = Recorded without detail　2 = Recorded in detail
   X = Not appropriate　　　　　　　　　　　　　　　　　　　　　☐

6. Occupational circumstances
   0 = Not recorded　　1 = Recorded without detail　2 = Recorded in detail
   X = Not appropriate　　　　　　　　　　　　　　　　　　　　　☐

7. Current medication/allergies
   0 = Not recorded　　1 = Recorded without detail　2 = Recorded in detail
   X = Not appropriate　　　　　　　　　　　　　　　　　　　　　☐

8. Examination findings
0 = Not recorded   1 = Recorded without detail   2 = Recorded in detail
X = Not appropriate   ☐

MANAGEMENT/ADVICE GIVEN:

1. Treatment/referral/follow-up
0 = Not recorded   1 = Recorded without detail 2 = Recorded in detail   ☐

2. Self-care advice
0 = Not recorded   1 = Recorded without detail 2 = Recorded in detail   ☐

3. Accident prevention advice
0 = Not recorded   1 = Recorded without detail 2 = Recorded in detail   ☐

4. Health-promotion advice (smoking, alcohol, drugs, etc)
0 = Not recorded   1 = Recorded without detail 2 = Recorded in detail   ☐

5. Discussion about use of health services: GP/A&E
0 = Not recorded   1 = Recorded without detail 2 = Recorded in detail   ☐

Index